Handbook of
Clinical
Pharmacokinetic
Data

Dedication:

To my mother, Annie Jack, 'Till a' the seas gang dry ...'

Handbook of Clinical Pharmacokinetic Data

David B. Jack

M

First published by
MACMILLAN PUBLISHERS LTD, 1992
Distributed by Globe Book Services Ltd.
Brunel Road, Houndmills,
Basingstoke, Hants RG21 2XS

ISBN 0-333-44489-2

A catalogue record for this book is available from
The British Library.

While every care has been taken in compiling the
information contained in this publication, the publishers
and author accept no responsibility for any errors or
omissions.

Typeset and printed in Great Britain.

Contents

Introduction

Collections of drug data are useful. One of the earliest I remember using was at the back of Smith and Rawlins's *Variability in Human Drug Response*[1]. I referred to it almost weekly, often wishing it were longer and more comprehensive. Since then a number of other collections have appeared, usually as appendices to works on clinical pharmacology and pharmacokinetics[2, 3].

For some time we have needed a pocket collection of pharmacokinetic data and I was pleased to accept the invitation to produce one. I use the word 'produce' intentionally, since there is precious little writing involved although there is a great deal of searching and evaluating. I have gathered data from research papers devoted to single drugs, reviews and larger collections of data.

About halfway through the preparation of this book an excellent little volume from ADIS Press[4] appeared and I was gratified and greatly encouraged by the measure of agreement between those data and my own.

The material gathered in the present volume should be of use to a variety of people including medicinal chemists, pharmacists, pharmacologists, clinicians, trialists and toxicologists. It can be used for theoretical as well as practical purposes.

Every effort has been made to make it as up to date as possible while still retaining data on older drugs and those compounds that are no longer used clinically but may still be of use in the laboratory, e.g. benoxaprofen, phenacetin, phenylbutazone and glutethimide.

The use of the individual entries and how they have been constructed is explained below and, in order to keep the size of the book small, compromises inevitably have had to be made.

A collection such as this owes a tremendous debt to the individual researchers who toiled to produce the original data and their efforts are gratefully acknowledged. Some so-called 'pure' pharmacologists sneer at the work of pharmacokineticists, toiling away to obtain clearance, protein-binding and other data on Drug A, publishing it, then starting all over again on Drug B.

However if you believe, as I do, that many scientific observations are only tiny pieces of a mosaic whose significance can only be seen when taken as a whole, then their efforts are worth while. The ultimate aim of pharmacokinetics is to allow drugs to be prescribed more safely and effectively. It never seems to occur to many of those 'pure' pharmacologists that the study of Drug X in a preparation of cockroach salivary gland (to take an example almost at random), to be followed by a study of

Drug Y under similar conditions, is not all that different in principle, except that pharmacokineticists are much nearer the patient. You can easily find cockroaches in hospitals — I know because I have worked in some — but none has ever to my knowledge been admitted as a patient.

At the very start I took the decision to rely only on published data rather than request material from the files of pharmaceutical companies, since the former have at least been subjected to peer review. When one begins to compile a work like this, it soon becomes apparent how few published data there are on some drugs, and for a number of drugs in the BNF no published data exist at all. These are, of course, drugs that reached the market a long time ago when regulations were less demanding; their use, however, has stood the test of time. Nevertheless, in order to use any drug safely and sensibly, we need basic data such as are gathered here.

Fortunately, new agents are now studied in greater detail than ever before and it is encouraging to see more pharmacokinetic studies in the elderly, using frail as well as healthy subjects, and in patients with renal or hepatic disease, in addition to those in young, healthy volunteers. More studies are also appearing examining the pharmacokinetic behaviour of drugs in other diseases such as spinal injury[5], burns[6] and cystic fibrosis[7], and at least one book has been devoted exclusively to pharmacokinetics in the elderly[8]. These advances are to be applauded.

I have produced what is essentially a 'pharmacokinetic' book, and the clinical data, by the very nature of medicine, are less precise. However, clinical material has been included to give essential background information and to complement the kinetic data. It hardly needs saying that, for reasons of space, the clinical material is given in only the briefest detail and the doses given in the tables should *not* be used to prescribe drugs. Texts such as the BNF itself should be consulted.

While every reasonable effort has been made to check the data, mistakes will inevitably occur and I should be very grateful if these were pointed out; I should also welcome suggestions for the inclusion of other agents.

The drugs have been set out basically according to the system used in the BNF, although one or two minor changes have been made. In a rapidly changing field such as clinical pharmacology this work should be regarded only as a 'snapshot' of the scene.

The selection of any piece of data requires that a decision be made and why should one choose a particular piece and not another? Take as an example the half-life of an intensively studied drug such as propranolol. If one were simply to search the literature and give a range that included all the half-lives that had ever been reported, the data would be of little help. Representative data should be chosen and outliers, for whatever reason, should be rejected. This is not difficult to do when one has a detailed knowledge of the drug in question, but very few of us can claim a really detailed experience of more than a few compounds. I have been forced to make many decisions throughout the book and I hope that I have been right most, if not all, of the time.

The Pharmacokinetic Tables

Physicians seeking to treat diseases and conditions with drugs attempt to produce appropriate concentrations at the relevant sites in the body for suitable periods of time. These periods may be relatively short, as in the case of many microbial infections, or for life, as in the case of diseases such as Parkinson's or hypertension. We now have a large measure of control over the rate at which we can deliver a drug to the body but this is useless unless we know in detail how rapidly and in what way the drug is cleared by the body. Only by balancing the rate of entry with the rate of exit can we obtain a desired drug concentration in the body. Today many pharmacokinetic models are more physiological than was previously the case[9] and this is surely a good thing. However, irrespective of the model used, we need reliable pharmacokinetic data. The individual parameters listed in the tables in this handbook will now be discussed in order to describe their usefulness and how they were obtained.

The first two parameters deal with the more chemical properties of a drug and quantify its dissociation constant and partition coefficient. This type of data and other related material, such as solubility, physical properties, etc., can be found in a number of the standard reference sources[10-14].

pK_a

Many, if not most, drugs contain acidic or basic groups capable of ionization, and the pK_a is an expression of the strength of each group: for an acidic drug, a low pK_a means that it is a strong acid, while the reverse is true for a base. The Henderson-Hasselbalch equation, for an acid

$$\log (\text{ionized/un-ionized}) = \text{pH} - \text{p}K_a$$

and for a base

$$\log (\text{ionized/un-ionized}) = \text{p}K_a - \text{pH}$$

can be used to calculate the degree of ionization of a particular group at a given pH and help predict whether a drug will easily cross membranes to be absorbed, metabolized or excreted. Drugs cross membranes more readily in their un-ionized forms. Many drugs contain more than one ionizable group, however, and in such cases prediction is more difficult.

log *P*

The partition coefficient, *P*, of a drug is a measure of its ability to distribute between a lipid and an aqueous phase when the drug is in its completely un-ionized state. This is largely a theoretical concept, since many drugs are ionized at all pH values encountered in the human body. The distribution coefficient or apparent partition coefficient, *P′*, measures the distribution between phases when the drug is ionized and is of more practical value.

Since a drug is at its most lipid-soluble when completely un-ionized, *P* will always be greater than *P′*. The greater the value of *P′* the more lipid-soluble the drug, and this can be of value, particularly within a closely related series of compounds. The more lipid-soluble will have better tissue penetration, particularly into fat and the CNS, and will be more readily metabolized, and little will be excreted in the urine unchanged. However, care must be taken when comparing distribution coefficient data from different sources, since *P′* values are very dependent on the lipid phase (often, but not always, octan-1-ol), the pH of the aqueous phase (often, but not always, 7.4), the temperature and the technique used.

P or, strictly speaking, log *P* values can be obtained from theoretical calculations for many drugs and these data are readily available[15, 16]. There are, however, a number of frequently used drugs, e.g. gentamicin, for which we do not have sufficient data to allow such calculations to be made. In this handbook, when calculated values are given, 'C' appears alongside. Otherwise, it can be assumed that the logarithm of the observed distribution coefficient has been used. Studies measuring *P′* values for different groups of drugs under carefully controlled conditions appear at intervals[17-20], but many more are needed.

Oral Absorption

The majority of drugs are given by mouth and the degree of absorption may vary greatly, depending on the nature of the drug. It is important to know how much of a dose is absorbed orally, especially in a study where different drugs are being compared. Absorption can also be affected by a number of factors, including the administration of other drugs, food and liquids, the nature of the disease or condition and the type of formulation. In order to keep the tables to a manageable size this type of data has been omitted but authoritative reviews are available and are frequently updated[21, 22]. Prediction of absorption is difficult, since there is still much we do not understand.

Bioavailability

A drug may be poorly absorbed because of its intrinsic properties or poor formulation, and, even when it is well absorbed orally, it may be inactivated by the mucosa of the stomach and metabolized in the small intestine or during its passage through the liver before reaching the general circulation. The bioavailability measures the actual amount that reaches the systemic circulation following oral dosing, and is expressed in the tables as a percentage of the administered dose (it can also be expressed as a fraction of the dose). Drugs such as glyceryltrinitrate, which are completely inactivated following oral dosing, exhibit zero bioavailability and must be given by another route. A list of substances with recognized critical bioavailability (listed by the German Health Authorities[23]) is given below.

Table 1 Drugs with critical bioavailability

acetyldigoxin	oral iron salts
allopurinol	isosorbide dinitrate
amitriptyline	isosorbide mononitrate
amoxicillin	levodopa
ampicillin	levothyroxine derivatives
atenolol	methotrexate
benzbromarone	metipranolol
bupranolol	metoprolol
carbamazepine	metronidazole
chlorthalidone	miconazole
clenbuterol	molsidomine
clindamycin	nicergoline
clomipramine	nifedipine
cyclophosphamide	phenoxymethylpenicillin
dexamethasone	pindolol
diclofenac	pirenzepine
digitoxin	prednisolone
digoxin	propafenone
dihydroergotamine	propranolol
dihydroergotamine	rifampicin
tartrate	salbutamol
disopyramide	spironolactone
doxycycline	terbutaline
erythromycin	tetracycline
fenoterol	theophylline
fluphenazine	triamterene
frusemide	trimethoprim
glibenclamide	valproic acid
glyceryl trinitrate	verapamil
griseofulvin	

T_{max}

This is a measure of the time taken for the maximum blood or plasma concentration to be reached after oral dosing: it shows how quickly a drug is absorbed. For many drugs this is usually of the order of 2-4 h but can vary greatly between individuals and is affected by factors such as food, other drugs and formulation. The values quoted here relate to the standard formulation taken in the fasting state.

V_d

The apparent volume of distribution is a measure of the extent to which a drug distributes itself in the body once it has been absorbed. Drugs with a low V_d are usually confined to the circulating plasma, largely owing to protein-binding, while drugs with a very high volume of distribution are usually taken up and retained by some tissue from which they are released only slowly. As a rule of thumb the following table might be useful.

Table 2 Apparent volume of distribution

V_d (l/kg)	Explanation
0.10	highly protein-bound
0.27	confined to extracellular fluid
0.40	reaches intracellular fluid
0.53	distributed in total body water
< 1	tissue sequestration

The apparent volume of distribution is sensitive to the effects of other drugs, as well as physiological and pathological states, and change in V_d is a good indicator of shifts of drug between tissue and other compartments. In the tables no attempt has been made to distinguish between $V_{d,ss}$ and $V_{d,area}$, although the former is better, since it is independent of changes in the rate constant of elimination.

Protein-binding

A number of drugs such as salicylate bind to plasma proteins, usually albumin. Many basic drugs (e.g. felodipine) bind to alpha-1-acid glycoprotein and some drugs even bind to enzymes (e.g. acetazolamide to carbonic anhydrase). This is important, since only the free (i.e. unbound) fraction of a drug is able to cross membranes and act on receptors; the equilibrium between bound and free is a dynamic one, however. Protein-binding is competitive and concomitant administration of other drugs may lead to a displacement of the equilibrium and alter the steady-state; disease can also change the amounts of albumin (e.g. renal or hepatic failure) and alpha-1-acid glycoprotein (e.g. myocardial infarction), and this can also affect steady-state concentrations of drug. It should also be remembered that albumin is present in tissues as well as plasma. For some drugs saturation of binding can be achieved at usual therapeutic concentrations but no attempt has been made to indicate this, because of reasons of space. This type of information is available in some of the larger texts[3].

Active Metabolites

These are important, since they may prolong the effects of the parent drug or they might be responsible for quite different effects. In some cases, what were identified as active metabolites have been developed as drugs in their own right (e.g. diacetolol from acebutolol or paracetamol from phenacetin). Renal function declines with age and the rate of elimination of metabolites is reduced. If no account of this is taken, by adjusting dosing schedules, then unacceptably high concentrations may arise. Where metabolism has been shown to be polymorphic this has been indicated.

$T_{1/2}$

This is a measure of the time taken for half the drug present in the body to be eliminated. It is used to calculate dosing regimens in order to achieve a required steady-state and can also be used to estimate the time needed to eliminate a drug from the body once dosing has ceased. It is usually calculated from the log-linear portion of the blood or plasma drug concentration-time curve. It can be used to detect changes in elimination due to changes in metabolism (such as arise from the stimulation or inhibition produced by other drugs or agents) or excretion (such as arise from changes in urine pH), and much of the older literature uses the half-life for this purpose; clearance is much better and modern studies determine both, as outlined below.

CL

The clearance is a measure of the volume (usually blood or plasma) cleared of drug in a given time. It is made up of renal clearance of the unchanged drug and clearance by other routes, such as bile or respiration; there is also metabolic clearance, usually by the liver. Because the half-life depends on the ratio between the apparent volume of distribution and the clearance, it *can* happen that a change in apparent volume of distribution is cancelled by a change of similar magnitude in clearance. Then no change in half-life will be observed even when something in fact *is* happening. For this reason both clearance and half-life are now determined in good pharmacokinetic studies[24]. Strictly speaking, clearance is a function of body size but is presented here simply in terms of volume cleared per unit time.

AU

This is the percentage of the administered dose that is excreted unchanged in the urine. It can be a useful guide to renal disease and of interest to the analytical chemist, who may wish a rapid qualitative means of testing for drug compliance. For many drugs that are acids or bases, with pK_a values within the pH range of urine, the amount excreted unchanged will be dependent on the urinary pH.

Chirality and Chronopharmacokinetics

Many drugs contain chiral centres and are capable of existing in different enantiomeric forms. A great deal of evidence has accumulated that the rates of clearance of these chiral forms differ, but for reasons of space no attempt has been made to indicate this in the handbook; however, a list of enantiomeric drugs which have been extensively studied is given in Table 3.

Table 3 Enantiomeric drugs studied in detail

acenocoumarol	metoprolol
carprofen	misonidazole
dextropropoxyphene	pentazocine
disopyramide	pentobarbitone
etodolac	phenprocoumon
fenprofen	propranolol
flurbiprofen	sotalol
hexobarbitone	tetramisole
ibuprofen	tiaprofenic acid
indacrinone	tocainide
ketamine	verapamil
ketoprofen	warfarin

The questions of chirality and its implications have attracted a lot of recent interest[25-27].

We also know that differences can occur in the pharmacokinetics of a drug, depending on when it is administered in relation to the natural rhythms of the body. This area of investigation, chronopharmacokinetics, is being actively studied, and a list of drugs at present claimed to exhibit such behaviour is given in Table 4.

Table 4 Drugs reported to display
chronopharmacokinetics

amidopyrine	hexobarbitone
amphoteracin B	indomethacin
ampicillin	ketoprofen
aspirin	lithium
carbamazepine	midazolam
cisplatin	nortriptyline
clorazepate	paracetamol
corticosteroids	phenacetin
cyclosporin	phenytoin
digoxin	propranolol
erythromycin	sodium salicylate
ethanol	theophylline
ferrous sulphate	valproic acid
heparin	

A number of reviews of our current knowledge in this area are available[28, 29].
Again, for reasons of space, no attempt has been made to address this issue in the
tables of the handbook.

The Clinical Tables

Dose

This is more or less self-explanatory. The information quoted, however, is really only a rough guide, since so many things must be taken into consideration in prescribing the appropriate dose of drug for any given patient. In general, the route is oral, and when another route is more usual, this is indicated. Dosing of some drugs such as neoplastic agents is very complicated and in such cases only the route is given.

Therapeutic Concentration

This is the concentration which needs to be reached for the drug to exert a significant clinical benefit without causing unacceptable side-effects. Again, it is intended only as a guide and actually in many cases we have no clear idea of the therapeutic concentration we need to achieve. It is worth remembering that we almost always measure the drug concentration in plasma or blood and the drug concentration at the site of action may well be different. At steady-state there should be a relationship between the concentration of the drug in blood and in tissue, but such data are not always available. In cases like this the maximum concentration after a standard single oral dose is given as a rough guide and this can be useful for the analytical chemist in choosing the appropriate technique to use. For the interpretation of clinical data more detailed and specialized texts should be consulted[30, 31].

CSF/Pl

This ratio is a good indication of the ability of a drug to penetrate the central nervous system. Generally speaking, within any closely related series of compounds the more lipid-soluble will show better penetration.

Milk/Pl

This is important because many modern drugs exert powerful pharmacological effects at low concentrations. Breast-feeding mothers can transmit substantial quantities of certain drugs to the neonate, whose ability to cope with foreign compounds is extremely poor. This parameter depends, of course, on the time of sampling of the breast milk in relation to drug administration, and guidelines for the carrying out and interpretation of such studies are available[32, 33].

T$_{1/2}$ in Renal and Hepatic Failure

These diseases may require alteration in the therapeutic regimen of certain drugs and this is indicated in the text: a '+' indicates an increase in half-life, a '-' a decrease and a '0' no change. In general, interpretation in the case of renal failure, or decline in renal function with age, can be related to creatinine clearance; no simple relationship exists for hepatic failure, which is multifactorial. Increased bioavailability can be observed in some cases of hepatic disease because of a reduced first-pass effect arising from shunting. It should be remembered, however, that in renal insufficiency, even if the drug itself does not accumulate, the metabolites will and these may be potentially toxic, as in the case of thiabendazole. A number of excellent reviews are available[34, 35].

Pregnancy Risk

Many drugs are known to damage the developing fetus, especially during the first trimester, which can result in congenital malformations. Some drugs also exert harmful effects during the second and third trimester, giving rise to retarded growth and poor functional development of certain tissues; some drugs are contraindicated throughout pregnancy[36, 37]. S/P means that special precautions are necessary and C/I means contra-indicated.

Drug Interactions

Entire volumes are devoted to this topic and here I have only attempted to give examples of the types of interaction that have been reported. The interested reader is referred to standard texts[38, 39].

References

Many drugs reached the market such a long time ago that little or no experimental work has been published relating to their pharmacokinetics. When no worth-while information at all is available, the drug is omitted. Concerning the data that do appear, we have, in general, attempted to give references that are as up to date as possible. Again, reasons of space require that a great deal of selectivity be introduced. For example, there are eleven different pieces of pharmacokinetic information alone in each table and, typically, these may come from six or seven different sources. To keep the references to a manageable number I have restricted myself to one relating to pharmacokinetic and one to clinical data for each drug. I hope not to have made too many mistakes in my choices. Inevitably, for some older drugs no new research data are available and reference has been made to work carried out many years ago.

Faced with choosing one from a number of references, I have chosen the most up to date that I judged suitable, on the assumption that this reference would cite the most important previous work. I must confess that I have not rigorously checked this assumption.

1. Variability in Human Drug Response. J Smith and MD Rawlins, Butterworth, London, 1973.
2. Handbook of Basic Pharmacokinetics. WA Ritschel, Drug Intelligence Publications, Hamilton, Illinois, 1986.
3. The Pharmacological Basis of Therapeutics, edited by AG Gilman, TW Rall, AS Nies and P Taylor, Pergamon Press, 1990.
4. Clinical Pharmacokinetics, Drug Data Handbook, ADIS Press, Auckland, New Zealand, 1989.
5. Clinical Pharmacokinetics 1989; 17: 109–129.
6. Clinical Pharmacokinetics 1990; 18: 118–130.
7. Clinical Research 1988; 36: 55A.
8. Gerontokinetics. WA Ritschel, The Telford Press, New Jersey, 1988.
9. Benchmarks: Alternative Methods of Toxicology, edited by MA Mehlman, Princeton Scientific Publishing Co., Princeton, 1989, pp. 37–58.
10. Analytical Profiles of Drug Substances, edited by K Florey, Academic Press, San Diego,

Vol. 1 (1972), latest Volume 18 (1989).

11. Martindale The Extra Pharmacopoeia, edited by JEF Reynolds, 29th edn, The Pharmaceutical Press, London, 1989.
12. Clarke's Isolation and Identification of Drugs, edited by AC Moffat, The Pharmaceutical Press, London, 1986.
13. Dictionary of Drugs, edited by J Elks and CR Ganellin, Chapman and Hall, London, 1990.
14. The Merck Index, edited by S Budavari, Merck & Co., Rahway, New Jersey, 1989.
15. Comprehensive Medicinal Chemistry, Volume 6, edited by C Hansch, Pergamon Press, Oxford, 1990.
16. Partition Coefficient, Determination and Estimation, edited by WJ Dunn III, JH Block and RS Pearlman, Pergamon Press, Oxford, 1986.
17. Journal of Chromatography 1976; 120: 65—74.
18. Journal of Pharmacy and Pharmacology 1981; 33: 172—173.
19. Reviews of Infectious Diseases 1988; 10: Suppl 1, S10.
20. Journal of Chromatography 1988; 452: 257—264.
21. Annual Reviews of Pharmacology and Toxicology, 1980; 20: 173—185.
22. Comprehensive Medicinal Chemistry, Volume 5, edited by C Hansch, Pergamon Press, Oxford, 1990, 1—43.
23. Drug Information Journal, 1989; 23: 429—438.
24. Pharmacological Reviews 1987; 39: 1—47.
25. The Lancet 1990; 336: 1100—1101.
26. Biochemical Pharmacology 1988; 37: 9—18.
27. Pharmacology and Therapeutics 1990; 45: 309—329.
28. Clinical Pharmacokinetics 1982; 7: 401—420.
29. Clinical Pharmacokinetics 1990; 18: 1—19.
30. Interpretations in Therapeutic Drug Monitoring. DM Baer and WR Dito, American Society of Clinical Pathologists, 1981.
31. Therapeutic Drug Monitoring. A Richens and V Marks, Churchill Livingstone, Edinburgh, 1981.
32. Drugs and Human Lactation, edited by PN Bennett, Elsevier, Amsterdam, 1988.
33. Clinical Pharmacokinetics 1990; 18: 151—167.
34. Journal of Pharmacokinetics and Biopharmaceutics, 1975; 3: 333—383.
35. American Journal of Kidney Diseases 1983; 3: 155.
36. Medical Journal of Australia 1988; 149: 675—677.
37. Medicine International 1988; 60: 2485—2488.
38. Drug Interactions. I Stockley, Blackwell, Oxford, 1991.
39. Drug Interactions. PD Hansten, Lea & Febiger, Philadelphia, 1985.

The Tables

The Tables

Pharmacokinetic data on anaesthetics and neuromuscular blockers

	pKa	logP	Oral abs %	Bio %	Tmax h	Vd l/kg	PrBd %	Met	T½ h	CL ml/min	AU %	Ref
Alfentanil	6.5	2.2	iv			0.7	90		1-2	330		1
Alphaxalone			iv			0.8	46		0.5	1400		2
Atracurium			iv			0.1-0.2	82		0.3	375-450		3
Baclofen		-1.4C	var		2				2-5	260	high	4
Bupivacaine	8.1	3.4C	iv			1.0	96		2-6	580	5	5
Etidocaine	7.7	3.2				2.0	94		2-3	1100		6
Etomidate	4.2	3.0				4.5	75		4-5	730		7
Fentanyl	8.4	4.1	iv			3.0	83		3	780		8
Ketamine	7.5	2.2	iv			2.0	12		3	1000		9
Lignocaine	7.9	2.3	good	35		3.0	60-70	+	1-4	350-1400	3-20	10
Mepivacaine	7.7	1.8				1.0	77		1-2	780	<10	11
Methohexitone	8.3	1.7C				1.0	73		1-2	830		12
Midazolam	6.2	3.7C	iv			1.3-2.2	>94	+	2-5	700-1700	<1	13
Procaine	8.1	1.9	good									14
Propofol		3.8	iv			5-25	93		3-10	1300-2200		15
Sufentanil	8.0	4.0	iv			2.0			2-3	730	<1	16
Thiopentone	7.5	2.6	iv			3.0	80		10	130		17
Vecuronium			iv			0.2-0.3	30-90	+	0.5-1	225-480	25	18

Clinical data on anaesthetics and neuromuscular blockers

	Dose mg/day	Ther conc mg/l	CSF/Pl	Milk/Pl	T½ RF	T½ HF	Preg Risk Trim	Drug Int	Ref
Alfentanil	0.03/kg iv					+			19
Alphaxalone	iv								20
Atracurium	0.5/kg iv				0	0		inhal anaesthetics	21
Baclofen	15-60		low						22
Bupivacaine	150 epidural	1-2							23
Etidocaine	400 infilt	1-1.5							24
Etomidate	0.3/kg iv								25
Fentanyl	0.05/kg iv							halothane	26
Ketamine	2.0/kg iv		+						27
Lignocaine	200 iv	1-6		0.4	0	+		diuretics	28
Mepivacaine	<1000 infilt	0.4							29
Methohexitone	40 iv	2-5							30
Midazolam	2.5-7.5 iv				0	+	3	alcohol	31
Procaine					+	+		acetazolamide	32
Propofol	2.5/kg	0.1			0				33
Sufentanil	0.08/kg iv								34
Thiopentone	100-150 iv							sulphonamides	35
Vecuronium	0.1/kg				0	+		inhal anaesthetics	36

References

1 Clin Pharmac 1987; 6: 275
2 Postgrad Med J 1972; 48: Suppl 2, 1
3 Anaes Analg 1986; 65: 743
4 Analyt Prof Drug Subs 1985; 14: 527
5 Clin Pharmacokinet 1987; 13: 191
6 Br J Anaes 1975; 47: 213
7 Clin Pharmacokinet 1987; 12: 79
8 Br J Anaes 1986; 58: 950
9 Clin Pharmacokinet 1987; 12: 79
10 Clin Pharmacokinet 1987; 13: 91
11 Br J Anaes 1979; 51: 481
12 Clin Pharmacokinet 1987; 13: 1
13 Anaethesiol 1984; 61: 27
14 Clin Pharmac Ther 1972; 13: 279
15 Postgrad Med J 1985; 61: Suppl 3, 64
16 Clin Pharmacokinet 1986; 11: 18
17 Clin Pharmacokinet 1987; 13: 1
18 Anesthesiol 1983; 58: 405
19 Med Lett 1987; 29: 59
20 Anaesthesia 1985; 40: 121
21 Anesthesiol 1984; 61: 328
22 Eur J Clin Pharmac 1991; 40: 363
23 Clin Pharmacokinet 1980; 5: 340
24 Eur J Clin Pharmac 1978; 13: 365
25 Lancet 1983; 2: 24
26 Eur J Clin Pharmac 1987; 32: 529
27 Drugs 1987; 34: 98
28 Clin Pharmacokinet 1985; 10: 1
29 Br J Anaesthes 1985; 57: 1006
30 Anesthesiol 1985; 62: 567
31 Anaesthesia 1986; 41: 482
32 Eur J Clin Pharmac 1983; 24: 533
33 Postgrad Med J 1985; 61: Suppl 3, 105
34 Br J Anaesthes 1987; 59: 1147
35 Eur J Clin Pharmac 1985; 28: 543
36 Anaes Analg 1985; 64: 212

Pharmacokinetic data on analgesic and antimigraine agents

	pKa	logP	Oral abs %	Bio %	Tmax h	Vd l/kg	PrBd %	Met	T½ h	CL ml/min	AU %	Ref
Amidopyrine	5.0	1.0				0.86	30		2-3	480		1
Aspirin	3.5	-1.1	good	low	0.25	0.15	70	+	0.3	650	<1	2
Benorylate		2.1	good	low				+			<1	3
Buprenorphine	*8.5	3.2C	good	c100	3	2.5	96		2-6	1200		4
Clonidine	8.2	1.6	good	50	1.5	2.4	20-40	+	6-25	3-12	30-50	5
Codeine	8.2	1.1	good	40	1-2	4-5	7-25	+	2-4	700-1600	6-16	6
Dextropropoxyphene	6.3	4.0C	100		2	3-16	70-80		3-24	1000	<20	7
Dezocine		3.6C	iv			9-12			2-3	3500		8
Diamorphine	7.6	1.0	good			3.5-5	20-35	+	0.05	1000-1400	<1	9
Diflunisal	3.0	4.4C	good		2	0.1	99		5-20	6-8	<5	10
Dihydrocodeine	8.8	-1.5	good	20	1-2	1			4	280		11
Dihydroergotamine	6.9	4.9C	poor	<5	0.5	6-23		+	2-4	500-1500	<5	12
Ergotamine	6.4	4.2C	poor	low	1-3	2			2	350-1000	<1	13
Fenoprofen	4.5	0.8	good		1-2	0.1	99		2-3	65	2-5	14
Ibuprofen	4.4	3.7C	100		1-2	0.1	99		2	60	<10	15
Levorphanol	9.2	3.4C			1-2	10	40		15-30			16
Mefenamic acid	4.2	5.3C	good		2		99		3-4		<50	17
Meptazinol	*8.7	3.8C	c100	2-19	1-2	5	27		2	2100	<5	18
Methadone	8.3	2.1	good		4	5	80-90		10-25	140	30	19
Methysergide	6.6	2.1C							10		56	20
Morphine	*7.9	0.2C	c60	c50	1	3.5	35	+	2.5	1200	10-15	21
Nalbuphine		1.1C	good		2-4				3.5-5			22
Naproxen	4.2	1.5`	c100		1-3	0.1	99		10-20	5	<10	23
Nefopam	9.2	3.7C			1-3		71-76		3-8		<5	24
Paracetamol	9.5	0.5C	good	80	1	1	low	+	1.5-3	350	<5	25
Pentazocine	*8.5	2.0	good	20	1	5-6	60-70		2-4	1250	10	26
Pethidine	8.7	1.6	good	56	2	4	40-70	+	3-10	600-1000	5-10	27
Pizotifen	7.0				5-7				26			28

* = more than one ionizable group

Clinical data on analgesics and antimigraine agents

	Dose mg/day	Ther conc mg/l	CSF/Pl	Milk/Pl	T½ RF	T½ HF	Preg Risk Trim	Drug Int	Ref
Amidopyrine									29
Aspirin	1200-3600	20-100 SA			+		S/P	coumarin	30
Benorylate	4500-6000	120 SA					S/P	hypoglycaemics	31
Buprenorphine	0.6-1.6 sl	0.0005-0.0009					S/P	maois	32
Clonidine	0.1	0.001-0.002		avoid				antihypertensives	33
Codeine	120-240	0.1-0.2		2.2	0			maois	34
Dextropropoxyphene	260	0.05-0.75			+		S/P	alcohol	35
Dezocine	5-20 iv	0.005-0.02							36
Diamorphine	5-60 sc	*	low					cns depressants	37
Diflunisal	500-1000	60-180			+		S/P	anticoagulants	38
Dihydrocodeine	120-180	0.07-0.15					S/P	maois	39
Dihydroergotamine	3 im	0.0002-0.001					C/I	beta-blockers	40
Ergotamine	6	0.0001-0.001		+			C/I	erythromycin	41
Fenoprofen	600-1600	20-30			0		S/P	anticoagulants	42
Ibuprofen	1200-2400	20-30		low	0	0	S/P	salicylate	43
Levorphanol	1-2 iv	0.02							44
Mefenamic acid	1500	0.3-2.4		low	0		S/P	sulphonylureas	45
Meptazinol	600-1600	0.01-0.1							46
Methadone	15-40	0.05-1		0.5	+			maois	47
Methysergide	2-6	0.04					C/I	ergot alkaloids	48
Morphine	60-120	0.05		2.5	+		C/I	cns depressants	49
Nalbuphine	40-160 sc	0.015						cns depressants	50
Naproxen	750-1000	25-50		<0.1	0	+	S/P	beta-blockers	51
Nefopam	90-270	0.07-0.15						anticholinergics	52
Paracetamol	2000-4000	10-20		0.8,avoid	+	+			53
Pentazocine	100-300	0.05-0.2			0		S/P	maois	54
Pethidine	300-900	0.2-0.8			+	+	S/P		55
Pizotifen	1.5								56

* = metabolized to morphine ; SA = salicylic acid

6

References

1 Pharm Acta Helv, 1973; 48: 181
2 Clin Pharmacokinet, 1980; 5: 424
3 Scand J Rheumatol, 1976; Suppl 13, 9
4 Clin Pharmacokinet, 1983; 8: 332
5 Eur J Clin Pharmac, 1983; 24: 21
6 Arzneim Forsch, 1978; 28: 308
7 Drugs, 1983; 26: 70
8 J Clin Pharmac, 1979; 19: 205
9 Drug Met Rev, 1975; 4: 39
10 Drugs, 1980; 19: 84
11 Br Med J, 1985; 290: 1287
12 Clin Pharmac Ther, 1981; 30: 673
13 Clin Pharmacokinet, 1985; 10: 334
14 Drugs, 1977; 13: 241
15 Clin Pharmacokinet, 1984; 9: 371
16 Res Comm Chem Path Pharmac, 1983; 41: 3
17 Clin Pharmac Ther, 1980; 27: 292
18 Drugs, 1985; 30: 285
19 Clin Pharmacokinet, 1986; 11: 87
20 Headache, 1976; 16: 96
21 Clin Pharmacokinet, 1986; 11: 505
22 Drugs, 1983; 26: 191
23 Drugs, 1979; 18: 241
24 Drugs, 1980; 19: 249
25 Clin Pharmacokinet, 1982; 7: 93
26 Clin Pharmacokinet, 1983; 8: 332
27 Clin Pharmacokinet, 1982; 7: 421
28 Eur J Clin Pharmac, 1983; 25: 759
29 Drug Ther Bull, 1976; 14: 55
30 Clin Pharmacokinet, 1980; 5: 424
31 Rheumatol Rehabil, 1978; 17: 23
32 Br Med J, 1982; 284: 1830
33 Br J Clin Pharmac, 1983; 15: Suppl 4, 455S
34 J Int Med Res , 1983; 11: 92
35 Drug Ther Bull, 1983; 21: 17
36 Clin Anaesth, 1983; 1: 159
37 New Engl J Med, 1984; 310: 1213
38 Drugs, 1980; 19: 84
39 Br Med J, 1983; 286: 675
40 Ann Intern Med, 1980; 92: 387
41 Drugs, 1983; 26: 364
42 Curr Ther Res, 1987; 41: 17
43 J Int Med Res, 1986; 14: 53
44 Res Com Chem Path Pharmac, 1983; 41: 3
45 Curr Ther Res, 1968; 10: 592
46 Postgrad Med J, 1985; 61: Suppl 2
47 Br Med J, 1982; 284: 630
48 Br J Hosp Med, 1984; 31: 142
49 Ther Drug Monit, 1991; 13: 1
50 Drugs, 1983; 26: 191
51 Drugs, 1979; 18: 241
52 Drugs, 1980; 19: 249
53 Drugs, 1983; 25: 290
54 Drug Alc Depend, 1985; 14: 313
55 Br J Clin Pharmac, 1982; 14: 385
56 Drugs, 1972; 3: 159

Pharmacokinetic data on anti-gout and related agents

	pKa	logP	Oral abs %	Bio %	Tmax h	Vd l/kg	PrBd %	Met	T½ h	CL ml/min	AU %	Ref
Allopurinol	9.4	-0.6	good	90	1-2	0.6	<5	+	0.5-2	800	low	1
Aurothiomalate			im				95		550		60-90	2
Colchicine	* 1.7	1.0	good		1-2	0.7-2	30-50		1	600	5-17	3
Penicillamine	* 1.8	-2.5C	poor		2-3		90		2-6	1000	3-25	4
Probenecid	3.4	3.2	good		3-4	0.1-0.2	90		4-17	23	1-10	5
Sulphasalazine	* 0.6	4.3C	irreg		3	<1	>95	+	6-17		2-10	6
Sulphinpyrazone	2.8	2.3	good		1-4	0.06	98	+	3-5	23	<50	7

* = more than one ionizable group

Clinical data on anti-gout and related agents

	Dose mg/day	Ther conc mg/l	CSF/Pl	Milk/Pl	T½ RF	T½ HF	Preg Risk Trim	Drug Int	Ref
Allopurinol	100-600	1.4-2.6			+		S/P	anticoagulants	8
Aurothiomalate	50/week im	3-5		avoid	avoid	-	C/I		9
Colchicine	1-10	0.0003-0.0024			+				10
Penicillamine	125-1500	1.7-5.6			avoid		C/I	antimalarials	11
Probenecid	500-2000	20-150			avoid		S/P	salicylates	12
Sulphasalazine	1500-3000	5-45		avoid			3	digoxin	13
Sulphinpyrazone	100-600	6-17			avoid		S/P	hypoglycaemics	14

References

1 Clin Pharmacokinet 1986; 11: 343
2 Clin Pharmacokinet 1986; 11: 133
3 Eur J Drug Met Pharmacokinet 1989; 14: 317
4 Clin Pharmac Ther 1981; 30: 404
5 Clin Pharmacokinet 1981; 6: 135
6 Clin Pharmacokinet 1976; 1: 406
7 Clin Pharmacokinet 1982; 7: 42
8 Br Med J 1987; 294: 1504
9 Med J Aust 1984; 140: 73
10 New Engl J Med 1986; 314: 1001
11 Arthritis Rheum 1982; 25: 111
12 Lancet 1976; 2: 376
13 Ann Intern Med 1984; 3: 377
14 Clin Pharmac Ther 1985; 37: 36

Pharmacokineic data on anthelmintic agents

	pKa	logP	Oral abs %	Bio %	Tmax h	Vd l/kg	PrBd %	Met	T½ h	CL ml/min	AU %	Ref
Albendazole		3.5C										1
Mebendazole		3.1C	poor		3-7	2	95		2-9		<10	2
Oxamniquine	*3.3	2.2	good									3
Piperazine	*5.7	-1.2	good									4
Praziquantel		3.4C	c80		1-3				1-2			5
Pyrantel	11.0		poor								5	6
Thiabendazole		2.3C	good		1-2				1		<1	7

* = more than one ionizable group

Clinical data on anthelmintic agents

	Dose mg/day	Ther conc mg/l	CSF/Pl	Milk/Pl	T½ RF	T½ HF	Preg Risk Trim	Drug Int	Ref
Albendazole	400-800	1	0.4						8
Mebendazole	100-200								9
Oxamniquine	15-30/kg								10
Piperazine	2000								11
Praziquantel	40/kg	1.6	0.2	0.3					12
Pyrantel	5-10/kg								13
Thiabendazole	50/kg				0			xanthines	14

References

1 Eur J Clin Pharmac 1986; 30: 705
2 Clin Pharmac Ther 1981; 30: 551
3 J Antimicrob Chemother 1987;
   19: 87
4 J Pharm Sci 1973; 62: 2024
5 Eur J Clin Pharmac 1978; 14: 281
6 J Pharm Pharmac 1970; 22: 26
7 Toxicol Appl Pharmac 1966; 9:
   31
8 Clin Neuropharmac 1990; 13: 559
9 Br J Clin Pharmac 1982; 13: 829
10 Trans Roy Soc Trop Med Hyg
   1987; 81: 55
11 Pharm J 1988; 240: 367
12 J Antimicrob Chemother 1985;
   15: 1
13 Med Lett 1986; 28: 9
14 Br J Opthal 1980; 64: 30

Pharmacokinetic data on antiarrhythmic agents

	pKa	logP	Oral abs %	Bio %	Tmax h	Vd l/kg	PrBd %	Met	T½ h	CL ml/min	AU %	Ref
Ajmaline	8.2	1.3C					80					1
Amiodarone	6.6	>7.0		60	2-8	12-70	96		50d	140-450	<5	2
Atropine	9.9	1.8	good		0.5	2-3	50		2-4	1000	50	3
Bretylium		<-1.0	poor	25	1-8	1-8	low		7-10	300-800	75	4
Disopyramide	8.4	1.4C	100	85	1-3	2-3	35-80		3-11	600	50-60	5
Encainide		3.8C	>95	55	1-3	2-4	70-80	+	2-12*	700	<10	6
Flecainide		4.5C				8	52		15	700	2-45	7
Lignocaine	7.9	2.0C	good	35		3	60-70	+	1-4	350-1400	3-20	8
Lorcainide		4.5C				10	85		9	1000	<3	9
Mexiletine	9.0	2.6C	>90	90	1-2	5-8	70		7-25	500	10-20	10
Moricizine		3.3C	100	36	1-2	8-11	80-95		2-4	1300-2700	<10	11
Procainamide	9.2	0.9	>95	85	1-2	2	15	+	3*	300-1000	45-60	12
Propafenone		3.2C	90	50		2.5-4	95	+	2-32*	1200	<1	13
Quinidine	8.8	3.2C	90	75	1	2-3	75-90	+	4-12	300	10-50	14
Tocainide	7.8	-0.1C	high		1-2	1-3	10-50		8-25	140-210	20-50	15
Verapamil		3.5C	90	20	2-3	4-5	90	+	2-7	700-1400	<5	16

* = genetic polymorphism

Clinical data on antiarrhythmic agents

	Dose mg/day	Ther conc mg/l	CSF/Pl	Milk/Pl	T½ RF	T½ HF	Preg Risk Trim	Drug Int	Ref
Ajmaline									17
Amiodarone	600-12000	0.5-2.5	low	avoid	0		2,3	warfarin	18
Atropine	0.3-3.0 iv	0.003		low					19
Bretylium	15.0/kg im	1-2			+			sympathomimetics	20
Disopyramide	300-800	3.0		avoid	+			beta-blockers	21
Encainide	75-200	0.02			+	+			22
Flecainide	200-400	0.12-0.80			+			digoxin	23
Lignocaine	100 bolus	5.0		0.4	0			diuretics	24
Lorcainide	100-400	0.15-0.40				+			25
Mexiletine	600-800	0.75-2.0		1.5	+				26
Moricizine	300-1500	0.5-1.7						cimetidine	27
Procainamide	1000	3-12			+				28
Propafenone	450-900	0.4-4.0			0	+		digoxin	29
Quinidine	800-1600	2-6			0	+		anticoagulants	30
Tocainide	1200	5-7			+	+		antiarrhythmics	31
Verapamil	120-480	0.25		0.6	0	+		quinidine	32

References

1 J Pharm Pharmac 1984; 36: 202
2 Clin Pharmacokinet 1984; 9: 136
3 Eur J Clin Pharmac 1984; 26: 613
4 Clin Pharmacokinet 1985; 10: 248
5 Clin Pharmacokinet 1986; 11: 214
6 Drugs 1987; 34: 519
7 Eur J Clin Pharmac 1991; 40: 155
8 Clin Pharmacokinet 1987; 13: 91
9 Clin Pharmac Ther 1979; 26: 187
10 Br J Clin Pharmac 1978; 6: 103
11 Drugs 1990; 40: 138
12 Clin Pharmacokinet 1978; 3: 97
13 New Engl J Med 1990; 322: 518
14 Clin Pharmacokinet 1980; 5: 150
15 Biopharm Drug Disposit 1990;
   11: 351
16 Clin Pharmacokinet 1985; 10: 248
17 Drugs 1981; 22: 363
18 Ann Pharmacother 1990: 23: 757
19 Br J Hosp Med 1985; 33: 138
20 New Engl J Med 1979; 300: 473
21 J Am Cardiol 1985; 5: 1457
22 Am J Cardiol 1986; 58: 74C
23 Clin Pharmac Ther 1990; 48: 262
24 Br Med J 1983; 286: 1332
25 Drugs 1984; 27: 29
26 Drugs 1990; 40: 374
27 Am J Cardiol 1990; 65: 26D
28 Clin Pharmac Ther 1984; 35: 285
29 Clin Pharmacokinet 1991; 21: 1
30 Am Heart J 1978; 96: 829
31 New Engl J Med 1986; 315: 41
32 Ann Intern Med 1980; 93: 875

Pharmacokinetic data on anticoagulant, antiplatelet and lipid-lowering agents

	pKa	logP	Oral abs %	Bio %	Tmax h	Vd l/kg	PrBd %	Met	T½ h	CL ml/min	AU %	Ref
Aminocaproic acid	*4.4	-3.0	good		2	0.4			2-5	190	70-80	1
Benzafibrate			good		2		94-96		2			2
Clofibrate	3.0	3.7C	c100	95	2-8	0.1-0.2	>95	+	12-25	10-20	15-30	3
Dipyridamole	6.4	2.1C	good	50	1	2.5	>90		12	140	<1	4
Gemfibrozil		3.9C	c100		1-2		97-99		1-2		50	5
Nicoumalone	4.7		good		2-3	0.3	>95		8	35	<1	6
Nicotinic acid	*4.8		c100		1				0.3-1		35	7
Phenindione	4.1	3.7C	good				70		6			8
Probucol		>10.0C	var								low	9
Tranexamic acid	*4.4	-1.9C	good	40					10	120		10
Warfarin	5.0	2.5	good		0.3-3	0.1-0.2	97-99	+	15-85	1.5-6.0	<1	11

* = more than one ionizable group

Clinical data on anticoagulant, antiplatelet and lipid-lowering agents

	Dose mg/day	Ther conc mg/l	CSF/Pl	Milk/Pl	T½ RF	T½ HF	Preg Risk Trim	Drug Int	Ref
Aminocaproic acid	12000-18000	100-400						antacids	12
Benzafibrate	600						C/I		13
Clofibrate	100-1500	100			+		C/I	anticoagulants	14
Dipyridamole	300-600	0.1-1.5			+			antacids	15
Gemfibrozil	300-1200				0		C/I		16
Nicoumalone	1-8	0.02-0.07					C/I		17
Nicotinic acid	300-6000	4-18						nsaids	18
Phenindione	50-150						C/I		19
Probucol	500-1000						C/I	hypoglycaemics	20
Tranexamic acid	4000-6000	10-50							21
Warfarin	3-9	1-3					C/I	sulphonamides	22

18

References

1 Aust J Pharm 1981; 62: 403
2 Eur J Clin Pharmac 1980; 17: 305
3 Clin Pharmacokinet 1978; 3: 425
4 Drug Intell Clin Pharm 1984; 18: 869
5 Drugs 1988; 36: 314
6 Br J Clin Pharmac 1981; 12: 621
7 Clin Pharmacokinet 1978; 3: 425
8 Eur J Clin Pharmac 1973; 6: 15
9 Drugs 1978; 15: 409
10 Eur J Clin Pharmac 1981; 20: 65
11 Clin Pharmacokinet 1986; 11: 483
12 Drugs 1985; 29: 236
13 Eur J Clin Pharmac 1981; 21: 209
14 J Am Med Ass 1985; 254: 2097
15 New Engl J Med 1987; 316: 1247
16 New Engl J Med 1987; 317: 1237
17 Br J Clin Pharmac 1983; 16: 491
18 Drugs 1984; 27: 148
19 J Paediatr 1975; 86: 459
20 Lancet 1981; 1: 450
21 Drugs 1985; 29: 236
22 New Engl J Med 1991; 324: 1865

Pharmacokinetic data on antidepressant agents

	pKa	logP	Oral abs %	Bio %	Tmax h	Vd l/kg	PrBd %	Met	T½ h	CL ml/min	AU %	Ref
Amitriptyline	9.4	5.0	good	50	2-4	15	91-97	+	8-51	850	<5	1
Butriptyline		5.1C	good		3		>90		20		<2	2
Clomipramine	9.4	5.2	c100		2-4	12-17	90-98	+	20-80	400-750	1-3	3
Desipramine	10.2	4.9	good		3-6	22	70-90	+	10-35	2200	<5	4
Dothiepin		2.8	good	30	3	70			11-40	2400		5
Doxepin	9.0	2.4	good	30		20	80	+	8-25	1000	<1	6
Imipramine	9.5	2.5	good	50	3-4	10-20	85-95	+	8-20	1000	<10	7
Lofepramine		6.5C	good	low	1		99	+				8
Maprotiline	10.5	4.2C	good	70	3-8	23-70	90	+	20-70	400-1400	<10	9
Medifoxamine					1	8-12			1-2	5000		10
Mianserin	7.1	4.3C	good	30	3	6-45	90-95	+	6-39	320	5	11
Nortriptyline	9.7	1.7	good	60	3-24	14-40	90-95		15-90*	660	<5	12
Paroxetine		3.4C	good	50	1-11		95				2	13
Protriptyline		1.2	good	90	6-12	22	95		c140	140-350	<5	14
Trazodone			c100		1-3		90-95	+	4-7		<1	15
Trimipramine		4.7C	good	40	3-6	20-50	95		10-40	700-1750		16
Viloxazine		1.3C	100		1.5	0.5-1.5	85-90		2-5		12-15	17

* = genetic polymorphism

Clinical data on antidepressant agents

	Dose mg/day	Ther conc mg/l	CSF/Pl	Milk/Pl	T½ RF	T½ HF	Preg Risk Trim	Drug Int	Ref
								As a class :	
Amitriptyline	50-100	0.1-0.2		0.8	0		C/I	antihypertensives	18
Butriptyline	75-150	0.024-0.11					C/I	alcohol	19
Clomipramine	30-150	0.1-0.5		1.0			C/I	barbiturates	20
Desipramine	75-200	0.02-0.88			0		C/I	maois	21
Dothiepin	75-150	0.02-0.06					C/I	sympathomimetics	22
Doxepin	30-300	0.05-0.15			0		C/I	phenytoin	23
Imipramine	75-200	0.01-0.11			0		C/I	and other	24
Lofepramine	140-210	c 0.003					C/I	antidepressants	25
Maprotiline	25-150	0.05-0.25					C/I		26
Medifoxamine	200-1000	0.2-1.4							27
Mianserin	30-200	0.03-0.09					C/I		28
Nortriptyline	20-100	0.03-0.34			0		C/I		29
Paroxetine	20	0.008-0.05			+				30
Protriptyline	15-60	0.11-0.38			0		C/I		31
Trazodone	200-600	c 0.7		0.14			C/I		32
Trimipramine	75-300	0.01-0.24					C/I		33
Viloxazine	300-400	c 1.3					C/I		34

References

1 Clin Pharmacokinet 1985; 10: 257
2 Arzneim Forsch 1974; 24: 93
3 Clin Pharmacokinet 1991; 20: 447
4 Am J Psychiat 1985; 142: 155
5 Clin Pharmacokinet 1983; 8: 179
6 Clin Pharmacokinet 1985; 10: 365
7 Curr Ther Res 1984; 36: 228
8 Drug Ther Bull 1983; 21: 99
9 Drugs 1977; 13: 321
10 Eur J Clin Pharmac 1990; 39: 169
11 Drugs 1978; 16: 273
12 Br J Clin Pharmac 1985; 19: 832
13 Drugs 1991; 41: 225
14 Drug Intell Clin Pharm 1983; 17: 736
15 Drugs 1981; 21: 401
16 Drug Met Pharmacokinet 1989; 14: 139
17 Drugs 1977; 13: 401
18 Clin Pharmacokinet 1984; 9: 261
19 Br J Clin Pharmac 1977; 4: 91
20 Drugs 1990; 39: 136
21 J Clin Psychiat 1984; 45: 3
22 J Clin Psychiat 1980; 41: 64
23 J Clin Psychopharmac 1985; 5: 102
24 Clin Pharmacokinet 1990; 18: 346
25 Br J Clin Pract 1986; 40: 59
26 Med Lett 1981; 23: 58
27 Hum Psychopharmac 1988; 3: 195
28 Br J Clin Pharmac 1983; 15: 263S
29 Clin Pharmacokinet 1979; 14: 129
30 Neuropsychobiology 1985; 13: 31
31 New Engl J Med 1982; 307: 1037
32 Drugs 1981; 21: 401
33 Drugs 1989; 38: Suppl 1, 17
34 Curr Med Res Opin 1977; 5: 217

22

Pharmacokinetic data on antidiabetic agents

	pKa	logP	Oral abs %	Bio %	Tmax h	Vd l/kg	PrBd %	Met	T½ h	CL ml/min	AU %	Ref
Acetohexamide		2.4	good		2	0.2	75-95	+	1-2		low	1
Chlorpropamide	4.9	2.3	c100		1-7	0.1-0.3	60-95		20-45	2	10-60	2
Glibenclamide	5.3		good		3	0.15	99		1-2	91	50	3
Glibornuride		3.0C				0.25	95		8			4
Gliclazide	5.8	1.5C	good		4	0.3	85-95		6-14	13	<5	5
Glipizide		1.9	c100	c100	1-2	0.2	98		2-6	40	3-10	6
Gliquidone		3.6C	good				99		1-2		<1	7
Glyburide	5.3	3.9C	good						10		<10	8
Glymidine		1.3C	>95				80	+	2-6		<1	9
Insulin			inact				5		0.3-2	150-600		10
Metformin	*2.8	-1.4	good	55	2	1-4	<5		2-5	500-750	30-50	11
Phenformin	*3.1	-0.8C				5	20		5**	750		12
Tolazamide	*3.5	1.8C	good		3		95		5-7		7-15	13
Tolbutamide	5.3	2.3	good		4	0.1-0.2	90-95		4-12	20	<5	14

* = more than one ionizable group   ** = genetic polymorphism

Clinical data on antidiabetic agents

	Dose mg/day	Ther conc mg/l	CSF/Pl	Milk/Pl	T½ RF	T½ HF	Preg Risk Trim	Drug Int	Ref
								As a class:	
Acetohexamide	250-1500	20-60			avoid		C/I	alcohol	15
Chlorpropamide	100-500	30-250			avoid		C/I	sulphonamides	16
Glibenclamide	5-15	0.17-0.36			0		C/I	oral anticoagulants	17
Glibornuride							C/I	chloramphenicol	18
Gliclazide	40-320	0.7-4.9					C/I	aspirin	19
Glipizide	2.5-30	0.11-0.49			0		C/I	salicylates	20
Gliquidone	15-180	0.7					C/I	diuretics	21
Glyburide	1.5-20						C/I	beta-blockers	22
Glymidine	500-2000					+	C/I	maois	23
Insulin	<80 units im						S/P	corticosteroids	24
Metformin	1500-3000	0.59-1.3					C/I		25
Phenformin							C/I		26
Tolazamide	100-1000	28			0		C/I		27
Tolbutamide	250-3000	50-100		avoid	0	0	C/I		28

References

1 Clin Pharmacokinet 1981; 6: 215
2 Eur J Clin Pharmac 1980; 18: 165
3 Clin Pharmacokinet 1984; 9: 473
4 Arzneim Forsch 1972; 22: 2153
5 Drugs 1984; 27: 301
6 Drugs 1979; 18: 329
7 Arzneim Forsch 1975; 25: 1455
8 Drugs of Today 1989; 25: 689
9 Arzneim Forsch 1964; 14: 394
10 Clin Pharmacokinet 1985; 10: 303
11 Br J Clin Pharmac 1981; 12: 235
12 Analyt Prof Drug Subs 1975; 4: 319
13 Drugs 1981; 22: 211
14 Analyt Prof Drug Subs 1974; 3: 513
15 Ann Intern Med 1973; 78: 541
16 Drugs 1981; 22: 211
17 Mayo Clin Proc 1985; 60: 439
18 Am J Kid Dis 1983; 3: 155
19 Drugs 1984; 27: 301
20 Clin Pharmacokinet 1984; 3: 473
21 Martindale 1989; 29th edn: 390
22 Pharmacotherapy 1985; 5: 43
23 Martindale 1989; 29th edn: 391
24 J Am Med Ass 1986; 255: 617
25 Can Med Ass J 1983; 128: 24
26 Br Med J 1977; 2: 1436
27 Am J Kid Dis 1983; 3: 155
28 Am J Kid Dis 1983; 3: 155

25

Pharmacokinetic data on antiepileptic agents

	pKa	logP	Oral abs %	Bio %	Tmax h	Vd l/kg	PrBd %	Met	T½ h	Clr ml/min	AU %	Ref
Acetazolamide	* 9.0	-0.3	good		1-3	0.2	90-95		2-13	45	70-100	1
Carbamazepine		2.5	c100	>70	9	1	75	+	18-65	16-64	<10	2
Chlormethiazole	3.2	2.4	good		0.6	3-12	60-70		3-7	700-1700	<5	3
Clonazepam	* 1.5	2.4	good	>80	1-4	2-4	85	+	18-45	70-100	<1	4
Diazepam	3.3	2.8	100	75	1-1.5	0.5-2.5	99	+	20-99	21-35	<1	5
Ethosuximide	9.5	-0.3C	good		3-7	0.7	<10		40-60	12	20	6
Lorazepam	* 1.3	2.5	good	95	1-2	1-2	90		9-24	70	<1	7
Methylphenobarbitone	7.8	2.0	<90	70	3-6	2-3	40-60	+	50-60	35	<2	8
Paraldehyde		0.7	good		0.5	1			4-10	140		9
Phenobarbitone	7.4	1.5	100	c100	0.5-4	0.5-0.7	50		c 100	5	25	10
Phenytoin	8.3	2.5	100		2-4	0.7-0.8	90		7-60		<5	11
Primidone		0.9	good			0.6	<20	+	3-20	35-50	15-65	12
Progabide	* 3.4	3.0										13
Valproate	5.0	2.8	100	100	1-5	0.1-0.2	90		6-20	7-21	<5	14
Vigabatrin		3.1C			2		low		5-7		c90	15

* = more than one ionizable group

Clinical data on antiepileptic agents

	Dose mg/day	Ther conc mg/l	CSF/Pl	Milk/Pl	T½ RF	T½ HF	Preg Risk Trim	Drug Int	Ref
								As a class:	
Acetazolamide	250-1000	10-15		0.3	avoid		S/P	oral anticoagulants	16
Carbamazepine	800-1200	4-12		0.4	+		S/P	maois	17
Chlormethiazole	320-800 iv	0.1-2.8				+		alcohol	18
Clonazepam	4-8	0.02-0.07					3	cns depressants	19
Diazepam	10-20 iv	0.1-2.5	yes	0.16	0	+	3	alcohol	20
Ethosuximide	500-2000	40-100		avoid	0	+	1		21
Lorazepam	4 iv	0.05-0.24	<1		+	+	3	alcohol	22
Methylphenobarbitone	100-600	2-3					C/I	alcohol	23
Paraldehyde	5-10 ml im	30-100							24
Phenobarbitone	60-180	2-30		avoid	+		C/I	alcohol	25
Phenytoin	150-600	10-20		avoid	0		1,3	coumarin type	26
Primidone	500-1500	5-12		0.2	+		C/I	alcohol	27
Progabide	1800								28
Valproate	600-2500	40-100		0.05	0		1	antidepressants	29
Vigabatrin	2000				avoid				30

References

1 Br J Clin Pharmac 1985; 19: 363
2 Clin Pharmacokinet 1978; 3: 128
3 Human Toxicol 1983; 2: 361
4 Drugs 1976; 12: 321
5 Clin Pharmacokinet 1978; 3: 72
6 Martindale 1989; 29th edn: 403
7 Clin Pharmacokinet 1981; 6: 89
8 Merck Index 1989; 11th edn: 919
9 Toxicol Appl Pharmac 1969; 15: 269
10 Analyt Prof Drug Subs 1978; 7: 359
11 Clin Pharmacokinet 1979; 4: 153
12 Analyt Prof Drug Subs 1988; 17: 749
13 J Pharm Sci 1982; 71: 633
14 Clin Pharmacokinet 1980; 5: 67
15 Br J Clin Pharmac 1989; 27: 19S-22S
16 Br J Anaesth 1986; 58: 512
17 Clin Pharmacokinet 1986; 11: 177
18 Eur J Clin Pharmac 1980; 17: 275
19 J Clin Psychiat 1986; 47: 238
20 New Engl J Med 1983; 309: 354
21 Neurol Clin 1986; 4: 601
22 Br J Clin Pharmac 1982; 14: 141P
23 Martindale 1989; 29th edn: 404
24 Am J Obs Gyn 1962; 84: 1778
25 Am J Kid Dis 1983; 3: 155
26 Drugs 1984; 27: 328
27 Am J Kid Dis 1983; 3: 155
28 Acta Neurol Scand 1984; 69: 200
29 Lancet 1986; 2: 511
30 Neurology 1987; 37: 184

Pharmacokinetic data on antifungal agents

	pKa	logP	Oral abs %	Bio %	Tmax h	Vd l/kg	PrBd %	Met	T½ h	CL ml/min	AU %	Ref
Amphoteracin	*5.5		poor			4	>90		360	28	<10	1
Bifonazole		4.8										2
Fluconazole												3
Flucytosine	*2.9	-1.7C	c100		2-4	0.7	low		4	13	>90	4
Griseofulvin		2.2	irreg			1.5			22			5
Itraconazole			c100	<90							<1	6
Ketoconazole	*2.9	4.3			2-3		99		6-10		<5	7
Metronidazole	2.5	-0.0										8
Miconazole	6.7	6.0C				20	92-99		24	760	<1	9
Natamycin		-2.9C	poor									10
Nystatin			poor									11
Ornidazole	2.3	0.6				0.9	<15		14			12
Terconazole		5.6C										13
Tinidazole	1.8	-0.3										14

* = more than one ionizable group

Clinical data on antifungal agents

	Dose mg/day	Ther conc mg/l	CSF/Pl	Milk/Pl	T½ RF	T½ HF	Preg Risk Trim	Drug Int	Ref
Amphoteracin	800	cl			+				15
Bifonazole	1% topical								16
Fluconazole				avoid			C/I		17
Flucytosine	2000	30-40			+		C/I		18
Griseofulvin	500-1000	0.3-1.3					C/I		19
Itraconazole	100-400				0	0			20
Ketoconazole	200-400	7			0		C/I		21
Metronidazole	1000-2000	1-3						anticholinergics	22
Miconazole	1000	1			0		S/P		23
Natamycin	7.5 inhal								24
Nystatin	1.5-4M units								25
Ornidazole									26
Terconazole									27
Tinidazole									28

References

1 Clin Pharmacokinet 1983; 8: 17
2 Arzneim Forsch 1983; 33: 745
3 Antimicrob Ag Chemother 1985; 28: 648
4 Clin Pharmacokinet 1983; 8: 17
5 Analyt Prof Drug Subs 1979; 8: 219
6 Rev Infect Dis 1987; 9: Suppl 1, S43
7 Clin Pharmacokinet 1983; 8: 17
8 Clin Pharmacokinet 1983; 8: 43
9 Clin Pharmacokinet 1983; 8: 17
10 Analyt Prof Drug Subs 1981; 10: 513
11 Analyt Prof Drugs Subs 1977; 6: 341
12 Chemotherapy 1976; 22: 19
13 Chemotherapy 1983; 29: 322
14 Antimicrob Ag Chemother 1969; 9: 267
15 Med Lett 1986; 28: 41
16 Curr Med Res Opin 1987; 10: 390
17 Eur J Clin Microb 1988; 7: 364
18 Drugs 1983; 25: 41
19 J Int Med Res 1977; 5: 382
20 Antimicrob Ag Chemother 1988; 32: 1595
21 Br Med J 1985; 290: 260
22 J Antimicrob Chemother 1986; 18: 213
23 Drugs 1983; 25: 41
24 Pharmatherapeutica 1983; 3: 441
25 Antimicrob Ag Chemother 1980; 18: 158
26 Br J Clin Pharmac 1985; 19: 211
27 Pharmacotherapeutica 1986; 4: 525
28 Drugs 1982; 24: 85

Pharmacokinetic data on antihypertensive agents

	pKa	logP	Oral abs %	Bio %	Tmax h	Vd l/kg	PrBd %	Met	T½ h	CL ml/min	AU %	Ref
Bethanidine	12.0		poor		2		<10		2-6		50-85	1
Cadralazine		-0.0C				0.7			3	180		2
Captopril	* 9.8	1.0C	75	65	0.5-1	0.7	30		1-2	900	50-70	3
Cilazapril		0.6	good	60	1-3	0.4		+	50-90	250	<1	4
Clonidine	8.2	1.6	100	95	1-2	2-4	20-40		10-25	3-10	30-50	5
Debrisoquine	11.9	0.8			2-4		25		3-30b		8-80	6
Diazoxide	8.5	1.2	iv			0.2-0.3	90		20-70	7	6-50	7
Dihydralazine												8
Doxazosin		3.8C							11			9
Enalapril	* 3.0	-0.1	good	50-60	1-2	0.7	50	+	35	600	17	10
Glyceryl tn		1.0C	good	low		3		+	<0.1	30000	<1	11
Guanabenz		3.0C	good		2-5	5-8	90		12-14	8000-17000	<1	12
Guanadrel		-2.2C			1-2		20		10		50	13
Guanethidine	* 11	-1.7C	poor	<50	3		<10		4-8d		25	14
Guanfacine			100	>95			20-30		15-17		30	15
Guanoxan	12.3	1.6C									5-90	16

Continued on next page

Pharmacokinetic data on antihypertensive agents (Continued)

	pKa	logP	Oral abs %	Bio %	Tmax h	Vd l/kg	PrBd %	Met	T½ h	CL ml/min	AU %	Ref
Hydralazine	*7.1	1.0		10-35	0.5	3-8	90		2***	3000	<1	17
Indoramin	7.7	2.3			3-4	7	70-90		2-8	140	<10	18
Isosorbide dn		0.0C	good	25	0.5	1.5	30-70		0.3-1	2500-4000	<1	19
Isosorbide mn		-0.4	100	90	1	0.6	<5	+	2-7	70-350	2	20
Ketanserin		3.0C	good	50	1		95		14		<1	21
Lisinopril	*1.7	-2.9	50	25-50	6-8				30			22
Methyldopa	*12	-2.6C	poor		3	0.6	<20		1-2	200-400	20-60	23
Midodrine		-0.4C						+				24
Minoxidil	4.6	1.4				3	<5		3-4	600	<20	25
Pentaerythritol tn		1.6C	poor				85		7			26
Perindopril		1.3C			1			+	3	500		27
Prazosin	6.5	2.2C		60	1-3	0.6	95		3	210	<5	28
Quinapril		1.8C						+	3			29
Ramipril		1.6C	good	55-65	<1		73	+	**1-5		<5	30
Reserpine	6.6	3.5C	poor				40-95		c 200	250	<5	31
Urapidil		2.7C	c100	78	0.5-1	0.4-0.8	75-80	+	2-3	120-240	10-15	32

* = more than one ionizable group   ** = metabolite   *** = genetic polymorphism

Clinical data on antihypertensive agents

	Dose mg/day	Ther conc mg/l	CSF/Pl	Milk/Pl	T½ RF	T½ HF	Preg Risk Trim	Drug Int	Ref
Hydralazine	50-100	0.1-0.2			+		1,2	tricyclics	49
Indoramin	50-200	0.08-0.22						maois	50
Isosorbide dn	30-240	0.02-0.1							51
Isosorbide mn	20-120	0.34-0.68							52
Ketanserin	40-80			+				antiarrhythmics	53
Lisinopril	10	0.04					C/I	antihypertensives	54
Methyldopa	250-750	1-5			+			maois,lithium	55
Midodrine	40								56
Minoxidil	5-10			0.8					57
Pentaerythritol tn	80-240								58
Perindopril	4	0.06							59
Prazosin	1-20	0.001-0.007						antihypertensives	60
Quinapril	5								61
Ramipril	5-20	0.001-0.005			+	+			62
Reserpine		0.0004-0.0006			avoid			quinidine	63
Urapidil	30-120	0.1-0.2	yes			+			64

* active metabolite

Clinical data on antihypertensive agents (Continued)

	Dose mg/day	Ther conc mg/l	CSF/Pl	Milk/Pl	T½ RF	T½ HF	Preg Risk Trim	Drug Int	Ref
Bethanidine	30-200	0.02-0.5					3		33
Cadralazine	30	0.25							34
Captopril	25-100	0.15		0.03	+		C/I	nsaids	35
Cilazapril	2.5	0.04			+*	+			36
Clonidine	0.15-0.3	0.0003-0.0004		avoid			3	CNS depressants	37
Debrisoquine	10-120	0.02-0.18						tricyclics	38
Diazoxide	300-900	15-50						diuretics	39
Dihydralazine	150								40
Doxazosin	8-16	0.008							41
Enalapril	5-40	0.04		+			C/I	lithium	42
Glyceryl tn	0.3-1 sl	0.001-0.002							43
Guanabenz	16-32	0.002-0.003							44
Guanadrel	400								45
Guanethidine	20-100				+		3	diuretics	46
Guanfacine	2-4								47
Guanoxan									48

Continued on next page

References

1 Clin Pharmac Ther 1975; 17: 363
2 Eur J Drug Met Pharmacokinet 1985; 10: 147
3 Clin Pharmacokinet 1985; 10: 377
4 Am J Med 1989; 87: Suppl 6B, 45
5 Clin Pharmac Ther 1981; 30: 729
6 Drugs 1985; 29: 342
7 Clin Pharmacokinet 1977; 2: 198
8 Clin Pharmac Ther 1985; 37: 48
9 Br J Clin Pharmac 1982; 13: 699
10 Clin Pharmacokinet 1985; 10: 377
11 Clin Pharmacokinet 1983; 8: 410
12 Clin Pharmac Ther 1980; 27: 44
13 Drugs 1985; 30: 22
14 Eur J Clin Pharmac 1979; 15: 121
15 Clin Pharmac Ther 1979; 25: 283
16 Xenobiotica 1972; 2: 35
17 Clin Pharmacokinet 1982; 7: 185
18 Xenobiotica 1990; 20: 1357
19 Clin Pharmac Ther 1985; 38: 140
20 Clin Pharmacokinet 1988; 15: 32
21 Drugs 1990; 40: 903
22 Eur J Clin Pharmac 1987; 32: 11
23 Clin Pharmacokinet 1982; 7: 221
24 Arch Int Pharmacodyn Ther 1979; 238: 96
25 Drugs 1978; 22: 257
26 Merck Index 1989; 11th edn: 1132
27 Drugs of the Future 1988; 13: 801
28 Clin Pharmacokinet 1980; 5: 365
29 J Clin Pharmac 1984; 24: 343
30 Eur J Clin Pharmac 1984; 27: 577
31 J Clin Pharmac 1985; 25: 633
32 Drugs 1990; 40: Suppl 4, 67
33 J Clin Pharmac 1978; 18: 249
34 Arzneim Forsch 1985; 35: 623
35 Br Med J 1985; 290: 180
36 Drugs 1991; 41: 799
37 Eur J Clin Pharmac 1978; 13: 97
38 Br Med J 1977; I: 422
39 Clin Pharmacokinet 1977; 2: 198
40 Int J Pharmac Ther Toxicol 1981; 19: 372
41 Am J Cardiol 1987; 59: 1G
42 Drugs 1986; 31: 198
43 Drugs 1987; 34: 391
44 Drugs 1983; 26: 212
45 Clin Pharmac Ther 1973; 14: 204
46 Clin Nephrol 1973; 1: 14
47 Am J Cardiol 1986; 57: 1E
48 Arzneim Forsch 1969; 19: 947
49 Clin Pharmac Ther 1980; 28: 804
50 Br J Clin Pharmac 1976; 3: 489
51 Drugs 1982; 23: 165
52 Drug Ther Bull 1984; 22: 7
53 Clin Pharmac Ther 1986; 40: 56
54 Med Lett 1988; 30: 41
55 J Pharmac Exp Ther 1976; 198: 264
56 Arzneim Forsch 1976; 26: 2145
57 Lancet 1977; 2: 515
58 Clin Pharmac Ther 1980; 28: 436
59 Clin Pharmac Ther 1990; 47: 397
60 Clin Pharmac Ther 1980; 27: 779
61 Eur J Clin Pharmac 1986; 31: 9
62 Curr Ther Res 1986; 40: 74
63 Clin Pharmac Ther 1973; 14: 325
64 Drugs 1990; 40: Suppl 4, 21

Pharmacokinetic data on antiinflammatory agents

	pKa	logP	Oral abs %	Bio %	Tmax h	Vd l/kg	PrBd %	Met	T½ h	CL ml/min	AU %	Ref
Alclofenac	4.6	2.5				0.1	>99		3			1
Aspirin	3.5	-1.1	good	low	0.25	0.15	70	+	0.3	650	<1	2
Azapropazone		1.0	good		4-5	0.2	99		8-24	7-14	60	3
Benorylate		2.2	good	low				+	1		<1	4
Benoxaprofen		3.2							27		<10	5
Carprofen		3.9C							13-26		<5	6
Diclofenac	4.2	1.5	good	55	2-5	0.15	>99	+	1-2	240	<5	7
Diflunisal	3.0	4.4C	good		2	0.11	99		5-20	6-8	<5	8
Etodolac		3.6C			1-2		99		7			9
Fenbufen	4.5	2.6	good		2	3	>99	+	10			10
Fenoprofen	4.5	0.8	good		0.5-2	0.1	99		2-3	65	3	11
Flufenamic acid	3.9	2.0					>90					12
Flurbiprofen	4.3	1.2	good		1-2	0.1	99		2-6	20	25	13
Ibuprofen	4.4	1.0	c100		1-2	0.1	99		2	60	<10	14
Indomethacin	4.5	-1.0	good		1-4	0.2-1	90-99		3-15	70-140	5-20	15
Ketoprofen	4.6	1.0	good		1-3	0.1-0.2	95		1-4	70-140		16

Continued on next page

Pharmacokinetic data on antiinflammatory agents (Continued)

	pKa	logP	Oral abs %	Bio %	Tmax h	Vd l/kg	PrBd %	Met	T½ h	CL ml/min	AU %	Ref
Ketorolac	3.5	1.9C	c100	90	0.5-1	0.2-0.3	>99		4-6	26-46	58	17
Lornoxicam					2-3				3-5		<1	18
Mefenamic acid	4.2	5.3C	good		2-4		99		3-4		<50	19
Mesalazine	*2.7	1.1C	90			0.2-0.3	43		1		<10	20
Nabumetone		2.8C		low			>99	+				21
Naproxen	4.2	1.5	c100		2-4	0.1	>99		10-20	5	<10	22
Oxyphenbutazone	4.7	2.7					99		45			23
Phenylbutazone	4.5	3.2				0.17	99		70	2		24
Piroxicam	4.6	0.3	good			0.1-0.2	99		30-60	2	10	25
Pirprofen		1.0	c100		1-2	0.18	>95		6-7	20-25		26
Salicylate	*3.0	0.1	good		1-2	0.17	85		2-30	10-60		27
Salsalate	*3.5	3.6C	good		1						<1	28
Sulindac	4.5	3.4	good		1		95	+	7		<20	29
Tenoxicam									37			30
Tiaprofenic acid	3.0	2.5C	good		1-2		98		1-2	75-100		31
Tolfenamic acid		5.7C				0.16	>99		2-3	155		32
Tolmetin	3.5	1.0	good		0.2-1	0.1	>99		1-6	70-140	<15	33

* = more than one ionizable group

Clinical data on antiinflammatory agents

	Dose mg/day	Ther conc mg/l	CSF/Pl	Milk/Pl	T½ RF	T½ HF	Preg Risk Trim	Drug Int	Ref
								As a class:	
Alclofenac									34
Aspirin	<8000	150-300SA						anticoagulants	35
Azapropazone	600-1200	34-54		low	+	+	S/P	phenytoin	36
Benorylate	4000-8000	120SA			+		S/P	methotrexate	37
Benoxaprofen	100	4			+	+	S/P	salicylates	38
Carprofen	50-100							antacids	39
Diclofenac	75-150	0.8-2			0		S/P	probenecid	40
Diflunisal	500-1000	66-183	low		+		S/P	uricosurics	41
Etodolac					0		S/P	corticosteroids	42
Fenbufen	600-900	8		low			S/P	spironolactone	43
Fenoprofen	900-2400	23-31			0		S/P	hypoglycaemics	44
Flufenamic acid	600						S/P		45
Flurbiprofen	150-300	9-17		low			S/P		46
Ibuprofen	600-2400	20-30			0		S/P		47
Indomethacin	50-200	0.3-0.6	+		0	0	S/P		48
Ketoprofen	100-200	6-14			+		S/P		49

SA = salicyclicacid

Continued on next page

Clinical data on antiinflammatory agents (Continued)

	Dose mg/day	Ther conc mg/l	CSF/Pl	Milk/Pl	T½ RF	T½ HF	Preg Risk Trim	Drug Int	Ref
Ketorolac	10	0.9		0.04	+	0			50
Lornoxicam	4	0.3							51
Mefenamic acid	500-1500	0.3-2.4		low	0		S/P		52
Mesalazine	2400	0.1-10		0.2					53
Nabumetone	1000				0		C/I	phenytoin	54
Naproxen	500-1000	23-51		<0.1	0	+	S/P		55
Oxyphenbutazone									56
Phenylbutazone		40-150							57
Piroxicam	20-40	9-16		avoid	+		S/P		58
Pirprofen	1200	20-40			+				59
Salicylate	20% topical								60
Salsalate	<4000	20			+		S/P		61
Sulindac	200-400	5			0	+	S/P		62
Tenoxicam	20	2							63
Tiaprofenic acid	600	19-73					S/P		64
Tolfenamic acid									65
Tolmetin	600-1800	8-79		<0.01			S/P		66

40

References

1 Clin Pharmac Ther 1978; 23: 414
2 Clin Pharmacokinet 1980; 5: 424
3 Eur J Clin Pharmac 1987; 32: 303
4 Br Med J 1973; 3: 347
5 J Pharm Sci 1979; 68: 850
6 J Pharm Sci 1980; 69: 1245
7 Drugs 1980; 20: 24
8 Clin Pharmacokinet 1991; 20: 81
9 Drug Ther Bull 1987; 25: 11
10 Drugs 1981; 21: 1
11 Drugs 1977; 13: 241
12 Analyt Prof Drus Subs 1982; 11: 313
13 Drugs 1979; 18: 417
14 Biopharm Drug Disposit 1990; 11: 507
15 Clin Pharmacokinet 1981; 6: 245
16 Clin Pharmacokinet 1987; 12: 214
17 Drugs Exp Clin Res 1985; 11: 479
18 Postgrad Med J 1990; 66: Suppl 4, S28
19 Curr Ther Res 1968; 10: 592
20 Clin Pharmacokinet 1985; 10: 285
21 Drugs 1988; 35: 504
22 Drugs 1990; 40: 91
23 Helv Chim Acta 1957; 40: 395
24 Analyt Prof Drug Subs 1982; 11: 483
25 Drugs 1984; 28: 292
26 Clin Pharmac Ther 1977; 21: 721
27 Drugs 1985; 30: 368
28 J Pharm Sci 1984; 73: 1657
29 Drugs 1978; 16: 97
30 Eur J Clin Pharmac 1990; 38: 547
31 Drugs 1985; 29: 208
32 Eur J Clin Pharmac 1985; 28: 573
33 Drugs 1978; 15: 429
34 Curr Ther Res 1970; 12: 551
35 Br Med J 1988; 296: 307
36 Eur J Clin Pharmac 1981; 20: 147
37 Br Med J 1984; 288: 1344
38 Rheumatol Rehab 1978; 17: 254
39 Clin Pharm Ther 1981; 29: 257
40 Drugs 1988; 35: 244
41 Drugs 1980; 19: 84
42 Curr Ther Res 1985; 37: 1124
43 Drugs 1981; 21: 1
44 Clin Pharmac Ther 1980; 27: 286
45 Curr Ther Res 1969; 11: 533
46 Drugs 1979; 18: 417
47 J Int Med Res 1986; 14: 53
48 Eur J Clin Pharmac 1990; 38: 343
49 Med Lett 1986; 28: 61
50 Clin Pharmac Ther 1986; 39: 89
51 Drug Exp Clin Res 1990; 16: 57
52 Curr Med Res Opin 1979; 5: 754
53 Drug Ther Bull 1986; 24: 38
54 Drug Ther Bull 1988; 26: 41
55 Drugs 1990; 40: 91
56 Drug Ther Bull 1984; 22: 88
57 Clin Pharmacokinet 1978; 3: 369
58 Eur J Clin Pharmac 1985; 28: 305
59 Drugs 1986; 32: 509
60 Br J Derm 1986; 115: Suppl 31, 63
61 Clin Pharmac Ther 1986; 39: 420
62 Eur J Rheumatol Inflamm 1978; 1: 3
63 Drugs 1987; 34: 289
64 Drugs 1988; 35: Suppl 1, 1
65 Acta Neurol Scand 1986; 73: 423
66 Rhematol Rehabil 1978; 17: 150

Pharmacokinetic data on antinausea and antivertigo agents

	pKa	logP	Oral abs %	Bio %	Tmax h	Vd l/kg	PrBd %	Met	T½ h	CL ml/min	AU %	Ref
Betahistine	*9.7	-0.1C	good		3-5							1
Chlorpromazine	9.3	3.4	good	25	3	21	95-98	+	7-120	630	<5	2
Cinnarizine	6.1C				2				5			3
Cyclizine	*2.4	4.0C			2				24			4
Domperidone	7.9	4.1		20	0.5						<1	5
Hyoscine	7.6	1.3	good	low	c 1	2			3	750	5	6
Meclizine	*3.1	7.0C										7
Metoclopramide	*7.3	2.6	>95	40	1-2	3	60-70		3-6	500-1200	10-25	8
Nabilone	6.5C		good						2			9
Perphenazine	*3.7	3.1	good			10-35		+	8-12	840-2600	1-2	10
Prochlorperazine	*3.7	2.4		<20	2-6	high			7			11
Promethazine	9.1	2.9	good	25	2-3	13	75-93		10-15	1100	2	12
Trifluoperazine	8.1	3.9			3-6				7-18		1	13

* = more than one ionizable group

Clinical data on antinausea and antivertigo agents

	Dose mg/day	Ther conc mg/l	CSF/Pl	Milk/Pl	T½ RF	T½ HF	Preg Risk Trim	Drug Int	Ref
								As a class:	
Betahistine	24-48						S/P	anticholinergics	14
Chlorpromazine	40-150	0.002-0.12	+		0	0	3	antidepressants	15
Cinnarizine	90	0.08					S/P	alcohol	16
Cyclizine	150	0.07					S/P		17
Domperidone	60-120	0.04	low	0.25			C/I		18
Hyoscine	1-2	0.0003		low			S/P		19
Meclizine	75-150						S/P		20
Metoclopramide	30	0.04-0.06		avoid	+	+	S/P	phenothiazines	21
Nabilone	2-4						S/P	narcotic analgesics	22
Perphenazine	6-12	0.0003-0.025					S/P		23
Prochlorperazine	10-30	0.0008					S/P		24
Promethazine	25-75	0.002-0.018					S/P		25
Trifluoperazine	2-4	0.001-0.004					S/P		26

References

1 Drugs 1983; 25: 77
2 Clin Pharmacokinet 1978; 3: 14
3 Drugs 1983; 26: 44
4 Analyt Prof Drug Subs 1977; 6: 83
5 Eur J Drug Met Pharmacokinet 1981; 6: 61
6 J Pharm Sci 1984; 73: 561
7 Martindale 1989; 29th ed, 456
8 Drugs 1983; 25: 451
9 Clin Pharmac Ther 1977; 22: 85
10 Curr Ther Res 1986; 40: 871
11 Br J Clin Pharmac 1987; 23: 137
12 Br J Clin Pharmac 1983; 15: 287
13 J Pharm Sci 1984; 73: 261
14 Postgrad Med J 1976; 52: 501
15 Am J Kid Dis 1983; 3: 155
16 Drug Ther Bull 1981; 19: 27
17 New Engl J Med 1968; 279: 596
18 Drugs 1982; 24: 360
19 Clin Pharmac Ther 1969; 10: 395
20 Arch Neurol 1972; 27: 129
21 Clin Pharmacokinet 1983; 8: 523
22 Drugs 1985; 30: 127
23 Drugs of Today 1978; 14: 120
24 Martindale 1989; 29th ed, 763
25 Br J Hosp Med 1984; 31: 354
26 Ann Intern Med 1980; 93: 284

Pharmacokinetic data on antineoplastic and immunosuppressant agents

	pKa	logP	Oral abs %	Bio %	Tmax h	Vd l/kg	PrBd %	Met	T½ h	CL ml/min	AU %	Ref
Actinomycin			iv						36			1
Aminoglutethimide		0.7	c100		1-4				9-16			2
Amsacrine	*8.2	2.9	poor		1		30		7		10	3
Azathioprine		0.1	good	>80				+	0.5		low	4
Azelastine		3.9C	90		4-5		78-88	+	25	90	10-60	5
Bleomycin			poor			0.35			4		1	6
Busulphan		-0.5	good						2-3			7
Carboplatin									120			8
Carmustine		1.5	good			3.3			0.2			9
Chlorambucil		1.7	c100		rapid			+	1.5	4000	<1	10
Cisplatin			iv				90		200	5	25-75	11
Colaspase			iv						8-48		<5	12
Cyclophosphamide		0.6	good	c75	1	0.70	20	+	2-16	70	<10	13
Cyclosporin			var	40		3.5	98		9-27	280	<2	14
Cytarabine	4.3	-2.1	<20		3-4	2.5	13		2-3	920		15
Dacarbazine	4.4	-0.2	poor				5		5			16
Daunorubicin	8.4	1.8	iv					+	19		50	17
Doxorubicin	*8.2	1.3	iv			43	71	+	30	400-1200	5	18
Epirubicin	*8.3		iv					+	40			19
Estramustine		4.9C	c75	75	1-3	5-63						20
Etoposide		-1.1C	c60	45			98-99	+	4-43	7-86	30-40	21
Floxuridine	7.4	-1.2	poor								low	22

Continued on next page

44

Pharmacokinetic data on antineoplastic and immunosuppressant agents (Continued)

	pKa	logP	Oral abs %	Bio %	Tmax h	Vd l/kg	PrBd %	Met	T½ h	CL ml/min	AU %	Ref
Fluorouracil	*8.0	-1.0	var			0.25			0.25	1000	<20	23
Flutamide		3.5C			1-4		94-96	+			<80	24
Hydroxyurea		-1.8	good		2							25
Ifosfamide			good		1			+				26
Lomustine		2.8	good					+			low	27
Melphalan		-0.5	var	var		0.5	50-60		1-2	520	13	28
Mercaptopurine	*7.7	-1.8C	c50	16	0.5-4		20	+	1-1.5		<10	29
Methotrexate	*3.8	-0.5C	good		1-2	0.8	50-95		4-10	200	50-95	30
Misonidazole		-0.4			1-7				8-12			31
Mitomycin	10.9	-0.4	iv								10	32
Mitotane		5.6C	<50								<10	33
Mitozantrone			iv						43		low	34
Mustine	6.4		iv						<0.05		<1	35
Procarbazine	6.6	-0.1C	good		0.5-1			+	0.2		5	36
Semustine		3.3	good								low	37
Streptozocin		-1.5	iv						0.5			38
Tamoxifen		6.6C			4-7				160		<1	39
Thioguanine	8.2	-0.1	poor					+	0.5-4		<1	40
Thiotepa		0.5	poor				99.7				<1	41
Vinblastine	*5.4	4.2C	poor									42
Vincristine	*5.0	2.8C	poor			8.4	75		23-85	128	<30	43
Vindesine	*5.4	2.4C	poor			8.8			24	300		44

* = more than one ionizable group

Clinical data on antineoplastic and immunosuppressant agents

	Dose mg/day	Ther conc mg/l	CSF/Pl	Milk/Pl	T½ RF	T½ HF	Preg Risk Trim	Drug Int	Ref
Actinomycin	1000	10-12	0						45
Aminoglutethimide	up to 1000							anticoagulants	46
Amsacrine	90-120/sq m								47
Azathioprine	1-5/kg	0.05-0.08			+			allopurinol	48
Azelastine	8	0.01							49
Bleomycin	10-60/w	0.15	0		+				50
Busulphan	2-4	0.05-0.13			0			cytotoxics	51
Carboplatin	400/sq m				+		S/P		52
Carmustine	200/sq m		good						53
Chlorambucil	0.03-0.1/kg								54
Cisplatin	<120 sq m/4w		0		+				55
Colaspase	100 u/kg iv								56
Cyclophosphamide	2-6/kg	1-6	0.5		+		C/I	sulphonylureas	57
Cyclosporin	14-18/kg			+	0	+		midecamycin	58
Cytarabine	2-4/kg	0.05-0.1	+	+	0				59
Dacarbazine	2-5/kg		low						60
Daunorubicin	30-60/sq m		0						61
Doxorubicin	20-30/sq m	0.01			+	+		methotrexate	62
Epirubicin	70-90/sq m					+			63
Estramustine	560-1120								64
Etoposide	50-100/sq m	1-20	+		+	0			65
Floxuridine	<30/kg		+						66

Continued on next page

Clinical data on antineoplastic and immunosuppressant agents (Continued)

	Dose mg/day	Ther conc mg/l	CSF/Pl	Milk/Pl	T½ RF	T½ HF	Preg Risk Trim	Drug Int	Ref
Fluorouracil	12/kg iv		+		0				67
Flutamide	750	0.05-0.18							68
Hydroxyurea	20-30/kg		+		+				69
Ifosfamide	<6000/sq m								70
Lormustine	100-130/sq m		+						71
Melphalan	0.2-0.3/kg				0				72
Mercaptopurine	2.5/kg					+			73
Methotrexate	10-25/w		low	c0.05	avoid		C/I	alcohol	74
Misonidazole	<5000/sq m								75
Mitomycin	2/sq m iv								76
Mitotane	6-15/kg								77
Mitozantrone	12/sq m iv		0						78
Mustine	0.4/kg iv								79
Procarbazine	50-300		+				C/I	alcohol,narcotics	80
Semustine	200/sq m		0		avoid				81
Streptozocin	1000/sq m/w		0		+				82
Tamoxifen	20-40							warfarin	83
Thioguanine	2-2.5/kg		0						84
Thiotepa	60 im								85
Vinblastine	0.1/kg/w iv		0		0				86
Vincristine	<0.8/kg/w iv		0		0				87
Vindesine	3/sq m/w iv		0						88

References

1 Clin Pharmac Ther 1975; 17: 701
2 Clin Pharmacokinet 1985; 10: 353
3 Drug Met Disposit 1977; 5: 579
4 Int J Derm 1981; 20: 461
5 Arzneim Forsch 1981; 31: 1184
6 Cancer Chemother Pharmac 1978; 1: 177
7 Clin Pharmac Ther 1983; 34: 86
8 Cancer Res 1984; 44: 1693
9 Clin Pharmacokinet 1983; 8: 202
10 Eur J Clin Pharmac 1984; 27: 111
11 Clin Pharmacokinet 1983; 8: 202
12 J Pharm Pharmac 1983; 35: 762
13 Clin Pharmacokinet 1991; 20: 194
14 J Clin Pharmac 1986; 26: 358
15 Clin Pharmac Ther 1971; 12: 944
16 Eur J Cancer 1972; 8: 85
17 Eur J Clin Pharmac 1985; 29: 127
18 Clin Pharmacokinet 1988; 15: 15
19 Cancer Treat Rep 1982; 66: 1819
20 Med Lett 1982; 24: 74
21 Human Toxicol 1986; 5: 136
22 Martindale 1989; 29th ed, 628
23 Clin Pharmacokinet 1983; 8: 202
24 Martindale 1989; 29th ed, 1400
25 Drugs 1984; 28: 324
26 Clin Pharmac Ther 1976; 19: 365
27 Clin Pharmacokinet 1983; 8: 202
28 Clin Pharmac Ther 1979; 26: 737
29 New Engl J Med 1983; 308: 1005
30 Clin Pharmacokinet 1984; 9: 335
31 Human Toxicol 1984; 3: 29
32 Clin Pharmac Ther 1983; 34: 259
33 Martindale 1989; 29th ed, 643
34 Cancer Treat Rev 1983; 10: Suppl B, 23
35 Br J Derm 1982; 107: Suppl 22, 25
36 Analyt Prof Drug Subs 1976; 5: 403
37 Martindale 1989; 29th ed, 649
38 J Clin Pharmac 1977; 17: 379
39 J Pharm Pharmac 1986; 38: 888
40 Cancer Res 1971; 31: 1627
41 Martindale 1989; 29th ed, 652
42 Clin Pharmacokinet 1983; 8: 202
43 Clin Pharmacokinet 1983; 8: 202
44 Clin Pharmacokinet 1983; 8: 202
45 Lancet 1984; 1: 1318
46 Med Lett 1981; 23: 71
47 Pharmacotherapy 1985; 5: 78
48 Diabetes 1985; 34: 1306
49 Drugs 1989; 38: 778
50 Cancer 1977; 40: 2772
51 Am J Kid Dis 1983; 3: 155
52 Cancer Treat Revs 1985; 12: Suppl A, 73
53 New Engl J Med 1980; 303: 1323
54 New Engl J Med 1987; 316: 521
55 Ann Intern Med 1984; 100: 704
56 J Pharm Pharmac 1986; 38: 264
57 J Clin Oncol 1988; 6: 1377
58 Med J Aust 1986; 145: 146
59 Br J Clin Pharmac 1979; 8: 219
60 Gut 1982; 23: A447
61 Sem Oncol 1984; 11: Suppl 3, 2
62 Eur J Clin Pharmac 1985; 28: 205
63 Cancer Treat Rep 1984; 68: 679
64 Practitioner 1984; 228: 725
65 Clin Pharmacokinet 1987; 12: 223
66 Lancet 1986; 2: 440
67 Eur J Clin Pharmac 1983; 24: 261
68 Drugs & Aging 1991; 1: 104
69 New Engl J Med 1985; 313: 1571
70 Lancet 1985; 2: 496
71 J Am Med Ass 1973; 225: 32
72 Ann Intern Med 1984; 101: 14
73 Clin Pharmac Ther 1986; 40: 287
74 Drugs 1990; 39: 489
75 Human Toxicol 1985; 4: 425
76 J Am Med Ass 1981; 245: 1123
77 New Engl J Med 1984; 310: 649
78 Ann Intern Med 1986; 105: 67

References *(continued)*

79 Arch Dis Childhood 1986; 61: 727
80 Lancet 1979; 2: 1249
81 Ann Intern Med 1980; 93: 286
82 Gut 1983; 24: A596
83 Pharmac Ther 1984; 25: 127
84 Scand J Haemat 1984; 33: 453

85 Can Med Ass J 1980; 244: 2065
86 New Engl J Med 1978; 298: 1101
87 New Engl J Med 1980; 303: 585
88 Drug Intell Clin Pharm 1980; 14: 28

Pharmacokinetic data on antiparkinson and related agents

	pKa	logP	Oral abs %	Bio %	Tmax h	Vd l/kg	PrBd %	Met	T½ h	CL ml/min	AU %	Ref
Amantadine	10.4	-0.4	c100		3-4	8			10-30	280	80-90	1
Biperiden		3.9C			1-2				18			2
Bromocriptine	4.9	6.6C	good		1.5-2	3	90-96		3	930	<5	3
Haloperidol	8.3	3.4	good	65	2-6	10-30	90	+	10-40	600-1300	<5	4
Levodopa	*9.7	-2.9C	good	33	1-2			+	1-2	1700	<1	5
Orphenadrine	8.4	1.5	good				20	+	14-18		<5	6
Pergolide		3.8C			1-2		90					7
Procyclidine		1.7	good	75	1-8	1			8-16	75		8
Selegiline		2.2C						+	39			9
Tetrabenzine					1-2			+				10

* = more than one ionizable group

Clinical data on antiparkinson and related agents

	Dose mg/day	Ther conc mg/l	CSF/Pl	Milk/Pl	T½ RF	T½ HF	Preg Risk Trim	Drug Int	Ref
Amantadine	100-200	0.1-1			+		S/P	anticholinergics	11
Biperiden	2-6	0.004-0.006							12
Bromocriptine	10-80	0.001-0.004			0			alcohol	13
Haloperidol	2-10	0.001-0.04			0		S/P	indomethacin	14
Levodopa	125-1000	1			0			maois	15
Orphenadrine	150-400	0.1-0.2						antihistamines	16
Pergolide	up to 5	1-2							17
Procyclidine	10-30	0.15-0.63						phenothiazines	18
Selegiline	5-10							pethidine	19
Tetrabenzine	25-200	0.015						maois	20

52

References

1 J Clin Pharmac 1977; 17: 704
2 Arzneim Forsch 1985; 35: 149
3 Eur J Clin Pharmac 1979; 15: 275
4 Int Pharmacopsychotherapy 1982;
  17: 238
5 Eur J Clin Pharmac 1980; 17: 215
6 Arzneim Forsch 1970; 20: 538
7 Neuropharmacology 1980; 19:
  831
8 Eur J Clin Pharmac 1985; 28: 73
9 Br J Clin Pharmac 1978; 6: 542
10 J Chromatogr 1981; 226: 175

11 Ann Intern Med 1981; 94: 454
12 Eur J Clin Pharmac 1984; 27:
   619
13 Ann Intern Med 1984; 100: 78
14 J Clin Psychiat 1983; 44: 440
15 New Engl J Med 1984; 310:
   1357
16 Lancet 1985; 1: 1386
17 Am J Obs Gyn 1986; 154: 431
18 Eur J Clin Pharmac 1985; 28: 73
19 Br J Psychiat 1983; 142: 508
20 J Clin Psychiat 1978; 39: 81

Pharmacokinetic data on antiprotozoal agents

	pKa	logP	Oral abs %	Bio %	Tmax h	Vd l/kg	PrBd %	Met	T½ h	CL ml/min	AU %	Ref
Amodiaquine		3.0	good		4			+				1
Chloroquine	*8.4	4.6	good	85	1-6	820	50-70		c40d	1080	c40	2
Dapsone		1.0							22			3
Doxycycline	*3.5	-0.2	c100		2	0.7	82-90		16-22	28	30-40	4
Hydroxychloroquine		3.7C	c100		3				3d		8	5
Mefloquine		3.4C	good		2-14	19	98		21d	30	5	6
Mepacrine	*7.7	6.2C	good				90		120			7
Primaquine		2.2C	c100		2-3	3-4	75-90	+	4-10		<5	8
Proguanil	*2.3		good		3	2.9	80-94	+	82		30	9
Pyrimethamine	7.0	2.7	good		2-4		80-94		3-4d	28	16-30	10
Quinine	*4.1	3.4	c100		1-3	2	70-90		4-15	90	5-20	11
Sulfadoxine		0.7C	good		3-6		85-90		3-8d		<50	12

* = more than one ionizable group

Clinical data on antiprotozoal agents

	Dose mg/day	Ther conc mg/l	CSF/Pl	Milk/Pl	T½ RF	T½ HF	Preg Risk Trim	Drug Int	Ref
Amodiaquine	1200	0.3-0.7					S/P		13
Chloroquine	500/week	0.02-0.2		2.9	+		S/P		14
Dapsone	200/week								15
Doxycycline	100	1.5-3			0		C/I		16
Hydroxychloroquine	1200	0.003-0.2		+			S/P		17
Mefloquine	250/week	0.4-1							18
Mepacrine	100							primaquine	19
Primaquine	15-45	0.13-0.18					C/I		20
Proguanil	100-300						S/P		21
Pyrimethamine	25/week	0.21-0.43		5.5	0		S/P		22
Quinine	1800	3-7	+		+		C/I		23
Sulfadoxine	500/week								24

References

1 Br J Clin Pharmac 1987; 23: 127
2 Br J Clin Pharmac 1987; 23: 467
3 Clin Pharmacokinet 1986; 11: 299
4 Eur J Drug Met Pharmacokinet 1983; 8: 43
5 Eur J Clin Pharmac 1985; 28: 357
6 Clin Pharmacokinet 1985; 10: 187
7 Toxicol Appl Pharmac 1978; 44: 225
8 Eur J Clin Pharmac 1986; 31: 205
9 Br J Clin Pharmac 1990; 30: 593
10 Pharm Res 1990; 7: 1055
11 Clin Pharmacokinet 1985; 10: 187
12 Analyt Prof Drug Subs 1988; 17: 571
13 Lancet 1985; 2: 805
14 Br J Clin Pharmac 1983; 15: 471
15 Lepr Rev 1983; 54: 139
16 Br J Clin Pharmac 1983; 16: 245
17 Antibiot Chemother 1962; 12: 583
18 New Engl J Med 1989; 321: 1415
19 Med Lett 1988; 30: 15
20 Br Med J 1985; 291: 23
21 Lancet 1983; 1: 649
22 Trans Roy Soc Trop Med Hyg 1975; 69: 139
23 Br Med J 1986; 293: 11
24 Chemotherapy 1969; 14: 195

Pharmacokinetic data on antipsychotic agents

	pKa	logP	Oral abs %	Bio %	Tmax h	Vd l/kg	PrBd %	Met	T½ h	CL ml/min	AU %	Ref
Benperidol	8.0											1
Chlorpromazine	9.3	3.4	good	25	3	21	95-98	+	7-120	630	<5	2
Chlorprothixine	8.8	2.7		40	4	10-20			8-12	1000-1400		3
Clozapine	8.0	4.3C	good	50	1-4	5	low		6-33		low	4
Droperidol	7.6	3.5					85-90		2-3		<10	5
Flupenthixol	7.8	4.5	good	55	3-6	12-17			14-36	500		6
Fluphenazine	*8.1	3.5	good		2-3		99		33			7
Fluspiriline	8.7	6.2C										8
Haloperidol	8.3	4.3	good	60	2-6	10-30	90	+	10-40	560-1200	<5	9
Lithium			100	100	2	0.8			27	25	c100	10
Methotrimeprazine	9.2	4.7	good		1-4	30			15-77		<1	11
Pericyazine		3.5										12
Perphenazine	*3.7	3.1	good			10-35			8-21	840-2660	1-2	13
Pimozide	*7.3	6.3C			4-8			+	18-48		<1	14
Pipothiazine		>12C									1	15
Prochlorperazine	*8.1	2.4		<20	2-6	high			7			16
Promazine	9.4	2.5										17
Promethazine	9.1	2.9	good	25	4	13	75-93		12	1100	2	18
Sulpiride	8.9				3-4	2-3			6-41	420	20	19
Thioridazine	9.5	5.9	good		1-4		>99	+	10-36		<1	20
Trifluoperazine	8.1	3.9			3-6				7-18		1	21
Zuclopenthixol	*6.7	5.7C										22

* = more than one ionizable group

Clinical data on antipsychotic agents

	Dose mg/day	Ther conc mg/l	CSF/Pl	Milk/Pl	T½ RF	T½ HF	Preg Risk Trim	Drug Int	Ref
								As a class:	
Benperidol	0.25-1.5						S/P	alcohol	23
Chlorpromazine	75	0.002-0.12	+				3	cns depressants	24
Chlorprothixene	60-200	0.01			0	0	S/P	antihypertensives	25
Clozapine	100-500	0.1-1							26
Droperidol	30-120						S/P	antidepressants	27
Flupenthixol	6-18						S/P	anticonvulsants	28
Fluphenazine	2.5-10	0.0002-0.004					3		29
Fluspirilene	2 im						S/P		30
Haloperidol	1.5-20	0.0008-0.033			0		S/P	indomethacin	31
Lithium	250-2000	0.6-1.2mmol/L			+		C/I	diuretics,nsaids	32
Methotrimeprazine	25-50	0.05-0.14					S/P		33
Pericyazine	15-30						3	alcohol	34
Perphenazine	12	0.0003-0.025					S/P	cns depressants	35
Pimozide	20-60	0.004					S/P		36
Pipothiazine	20 depot 4w	0.018-0.058					3		37
Prochlorperazine	25-100	0.0008					S/P		38
Promazine	100-800						3		39
Promethazine	25-75	0.01					S/P		40
Sulipride	400-2400	0.18-0.32					S/P		41
Thioridazine	150-800	0.05-0.5					3		42
Trifluoperazine	5-10	0.001-0.004					3		43
Zuclopenthixol	20-150						S/P		44

References

1 Martindale 1989; 29th ed, 714
2 Clin Pharmacokinet 1978; 3: 14
3 J Analyt Toxicol 1983; 7: 29
4 Eur J Clin Pharmac 1988; 34: 445
5 Clin Pharmacokinet 1977; 2: 344
6 Eur J Clin Pharmac 1980; 18: 355
7 Eur J Clin Pharmac 1983; 25: 709
8 Arzneim Forsch 1970; 20: 1689
9 Curr Ther Res 1977; 21: 390
10 Ther Drug Monit 1980; 2: 73
11 Clin Pharmac Ther 1976; 19: 435
12 J Pharm Sci 1974; 63: 389
13 Curr Ther Res 1986; 40: 871
14 Drugs 1976; 12: 1
15 Therapie 1986; 41: 27
16 Br J Clin Pharmac 1987; 23: 137
17 Martindale 1989; 29th ed, 765
18 Br J Clin Pharmac 1983; 15: 287
19 J Pharm Sci 1984; 73: 1128
20 Eur J Clin Pharmac 1978; 14: 341
21 J Pharm Sci 1975; 64: 1177
22 Acta Psychiat Scand 1981; 64: Suppl 294, 1
23 Drug Ther Bull 1974; 12: 12
24 Am J Kid Dis 1983; 3: 155
25 Pain 1978; 5: 367
26 New Engl J Med 1991; 324: 746
27 Martindale 1989; 29th ed, 735
28 Psychopharmacologie 1976; 27: 1
29 Lancet 1978; 1: 1217
30 Br Med J 1977; 2: 1541
31 J Clin Psychiat 1978; 39: 807
32 Clin Pharmacokinet 1980; 5: 385
33 Postgrad Med J 1984; 60: 881
34 Arzneim Forsch 1967; 17: 159
35 Drugs of Today 1978; 14: 120
36 Br J Clin Pharmac 1979; 7: 533
37 Br Med J 1984; 289: 734
38 Br Med J 1987; 294: 167
39 Med J Aust 1975; 2: 342
40 Br Med J 1985; 290: 1173
41 Drug Ther Bull 1984; 22: 31
42 Curr Ther Res 1977; 21: 720
43 Curr Ther Res 1977; 22: 635
44 Mol Pharmac 1974; 10: 759

Pharmacokinetic data on antispasmodic, antiulcer and antidiarrhoea agents

	pKa	logP	Oral abs %	Bio %	Tmax h	Vd l/kg	PrBd %	Met	T½ h	CL ml/min	AU %	Ref
Atropine	9.9	1.8	good		0.5	2-3	50		2-4	1000	50	1
Azathioprine	* 8.2	0.1	good		1		30	+	0.5		10	2
Carbenoxolone	* 7.1	1.3	>95		1-2	0.1	>99		8-20		<5	3
Cimetidine	6.8	0.4	>95	70	1-2	1-2	13-26		1-3	600	40-80	4
Codeine	8.2	1.1	good	50	1-2	3-5	7-25	+	2-4	700-1000	6-16	5
Dicyclomine		5.8C	95	90	1.5				5			6
Diphenoxylate	7.1	5.0C			2	4-5		+	2-3		<1	7
Domperidone	7.9	4.1		20	0.5						<1	8
Etintidine					1						37	9
Famotidine		-0.6	<100	43	1-4	1	16		2-7	240-1000	72	10
Glycopyrronium			poor						<0.1			11
Hyoscine	7.6	1.2	good	low	0.5	2			2-3	750	5	12
Loperamide	8.7	3.9C	poor	low	4-5		97		7-15		1-2	13
Mepenzolate			poor				10		7-14			14
Mesalazine	* 2.7	1.1C	90			0.2-0.3	43		1		<10	15
Metoclopramide	* 7.3	2.6	>95	40	1-2	3	60-70		3-6	500-1200	10-25	16
Nizatidine		-0.6C	>95	95	1-2	1.2	15-30		1.3	840	65	17
Omeprazole		2.2	good	70	<0.5	0.17	94-96		0.5-1	560	<1	18
Pirenzepine	* 8.1	1.2C	poor	25	2		10		11	240	20	19
Prednisolone		1.6	>95	80	1-2	0.5-1.3	65-90		3-4	100-200		20
Propantheline			poor	low					2	1300		21
Ranitidine	* 8.2	0.3	good	55	1-4	1-2	15		2-3	700	25-50	22
Roxatidine		2.7C			1						55	23
Sodium cromoglycate	* 2.5	1.9	poor		0.25		60-70		1-2	560	<5	24
Sulphasalazine	* 0.6	4.3C	irreg		3	<1	>95	+	6-17		2-10	25

* = more than one ionizable group

Clinical data on antispasmodic, antiulcer and antidiarrhoea agents

	Dose mg/day	Ther conc mg/l	CSF/Pl	Milk/Pl	T½ RF	T½ HF	Preg Risk Trim	Drug Int	Ref
Atropine	0.25-2	0.003		low					26
Azathioprine	1-3/kg	0.05-0.08			+			allopurinol	27
Carbenoxolone	100-300							spironolactone	28
Cimetidine	800	0.26-0.80	0.2	>1,avoid	+	+		anticoagulants	29
Codeine	60-360	0.11-0.23		2.2	0		avoid 1		30
Dicyclomine	30-60								31
Diphenoxylate	25	0.01						maois	32
Domperidone	40-120	0.04	low	0.25					33
Etintidine	300	2.1					C/I		34
Famotidine	20-40	0.01-0.1	<0.1	0.4-2	+			antacids	35
Glycopyrronium	3-12						S/P		36
Hyoscine	80			low					37
Loperamide	16	0.002							38
Mepenzolate	100-200			low				tricyclics	39
Mesalazine	1200-2400	0.1-10		0.2				lactulose	40
Metoclopramide	30	0.07-0.13		avoid	+	+		anticholinergics	41
Nizatidine	150-300	1-3			+				42
Omeprazole	10-90	1			0			disulfiram	43
Pirenzepine	100	0.05							44
Prednisolone	40 o,60 iv	0.65		0.13		+	S/P	nsaids	45
Propantheline	45								46
Ranitidine	300	0.31-0.82	<0.1	>1	+	+		antacids	47
Roxatidine	25-150	0.1-0.8							48
Sodium cromoglycate	800	0.006-0.012						maois	49
Sulphasalazine	4-80	7-32		avoid			3	digoxin	50

References

1 Eur J Clin Pharmac 1984; 26: 613
2 Int J Derm 1981; 20: 461
3 Drugs 1976; 11: 245
4 Clin Pharmacokinet 1991; 20: 218
5 Clin Pharmac Ther 1974; 15: 215
6 Br Med J 1985; 291: 1014
7 Clin Pharmac Ther 1972; 13: 407
8 Eur J Drug Met Pharmacokinet 1981; 6: 61
9 Clin Pharmacokinet 1991; 20: 218
10 Drugs 1989; 38: 560
11 J Pharm Pharmac 1974; 26: 352
12 J Pharm Biomed Anal 1983; 1: 363
13 J Clin Pharmac 1979; 19: 211
14 J Pharm Sci 1972; 61: 1663
15 Clin Pharmacokinet 1985; 10: 285
16 Clin Pharmacokinet 1983; 8: 523
17 Drug Met Disposit 1986; 14: 175
18 Eur J Clin Pharmac 1990; 39: 195
19 Scand J Gast 1979; 14: Suppl 57
20 Clin Pharmacokinet 1979; 4: 111
21 Br J Clin Pharmac 1977; 7: 89
22 Clin Pharmacokinet 1984; 9: 211
23 Clin Pharmacokinet 1991; 20: 218
24 J Pharm Pharmac 1972; 24: 525
25 Clin Pharmacokinet 1985; 10: 285
26 Br J Anaesth 1984; 56: 19
27 Lancet 1976; 1: 1213
28 Gastroenterology 1978; 74: 7
29 Gastroenterology 1985; 89: 532
30 Br Med J 1980; 280: 524
31 Br Med J 1985; 291: 1014
32 Br Med J 1971; 3: 105
33 Gut 1983; 24: 1135
34 Eur J Clin Pharmac 1988; 34: 101
35 Drugs 1986; 32: 197
36 Br J Clin Pharmac 1983; 16: 523
37 Clin Pharmac Ther 1968; 9: 745
38 J Am Med Ass 1986; 255: 757
39 Toxicol Appl Pharmac 1971; 18: 185
40 Am J Gastroenterol 1990; 85: 331
41 Eur J Clin Pharmac 1991; 40: 423
42 Clin Pharmac Ther 1990; 47: 724
43 New Engl J Med 1991; 324: 915
44 Drugs 1985; 30: 85
45 J Endocrinol 1959; 18: 278
46 Prescribers J 1984; 24: 106
47 New Engl J Med 1990; 323: 1672
48 Drugs 1988; 35: Suppl 3, 48
49 Gut 1981; 22: 55
50 Drugs 1986; 32: Suppl 1, 18

62

Pharmacokinetic data on antituberculous and antileprotic agents

	pKa	logP	Oral abs %	Bio %	Tmax h	Vd l/kg	PrBd %	Met	T½ h	CL ml/min	AU %	Ref
Capreomycin	*3.3		poor		1-2						50	1
Clofazimine	8.4		<90		4		<20		70d		<1	2
Cycloserine	*4.5		c100		2-4				4-30		65	3
Ethambutol	*9.5	0.1C	c80		2-4	2.5	10-40		10-15	50-600	50-90	4
Isoniazid	*3.5	-0.7	c100	80	1-4	0.6-0.8	<5	+	1-5**	200-500	5-30	5
PAS	*3.3	0.9	poor		1-2		58-73		1		50	6
Pyrazinamide	0.5	-0.6	good		1-2		50		4-10		4-14	7
Rifampicin	*1.7	2.4C	good			1	80	+	2-6	170	15-30	8
Streptomycin					1-2	0.3	50		3		30-90	9

* more than one ionizable group   ** = genetic polymorphism

Clinical data on antituberculous and antileprotic agents

	Dose mg/day	Ther conc mg/l	CSF/Pl	Milk/Pl	T½ RF	T½ HF	Preg Risk Trim	Drug Int	Ref
Capreomycin	20mg/kg im	30						streptomycin	10
Clofazimine	50-300	0.1		+					11
Cycloserine	25-1000	22-34	+	+	avoid				12
Ethambutol	1200-1800	3-6	+		+			alcohol	13
Isoniazid	<200	3-10		avoid	0	+			14
PAS	12000	1-2		+					15
Pyrazinamide	2000-3000	134	+	+					16
Rifampicin	600	0.5-10	+	+	0	+	C/I	anticoagulants	17
Streptomycin	1000 im	40-50							18

References

1 Tubercle 1972; 53: 47
2 Drug Met Disposit 1981; 9: 521
3 Arzneim Forsch 1972; 22: 1769
4 Clin Pharmac Ther 1977; 22: 615
5 Clin Pharmacokinet 1979; 4: 401
6 J Pharm Sci 1974; 63: 708
7 Tubercle 1976; 57: 97
8 Clin Pharmacokinet 1978; 3: 108
9 Analyt Prof Drug Subs 1986; 16: 507
10 Tubercle 1972; 53: 47
11 Ann Int Med 1982; 97: 788
12 Antimicrob Ag Chemother 1987; 31: 969
13 Eur J Clin Pharmac 1973; 6: 133
14 Tubercle 1984; 65: 211
15 Arch Intern Med 1984; 144: 1888
16 Tubercle 1984; 65: 1
17 Antimicrob Ag Chemother 1985; 28: 467
18 Br Med J 1970; 1: 614

Pharmacokinetic data on antiviral agents

	pKa	logP	Oral abs %	Bio %	Tmax h	Vd l/kg	PrBd %	Met	T½ h	CL ml/min	AU %	Ref
Acyclovir	*2.3	-1.7	20			0.7	9-33		3	200	40-70	1
Amantadine	10.4	-0.4	c100		3-4	8			10-30	275	80-90	2
Foscarnet						0.6-2			3-6	150		3
Ganciclovir		-2.8C		6	1-2	0.4-0.6	<5		2-4	200	>95 iv	4
Idoxuridine							low				low	5
Vidarabine	*3.5	-1.2						+	3-4		1-3	6
Zidovudine			c100	60	0.5-2	1.4	<25	+	1-2	1600	57-72	7

* = more than one ionizable group

Clinical data on antiviral agents

	Dose mg/day	Ther conc mg/l	CSF/Pl	Milk/Pl	T½ RF	T½ HF	Preg Risk Trim	Drug Int	Ref
Acyclovir	1000-2000	10		avoid	+			probenecid	8
Amantadine	100-200	0.1-1.0	+	+	+			anticholinergics	9
Foscarnet	c 0.1/kg/min						S/P	pentamidine	10
Ganciclovir	5-10/kg iv	20-45umol/L	0.7	+					11
Idoxuridine	0.1% topical								12
Vidarabine	10/kg iv	0.4			+		S/P		13
Zidovudine	1200-1800		c1.0				S/P		14

References

1 J Antimicrob Chemother 1983; 12: SupplB 29
2 Ann Int Med 1981; 94: 454
3 Antimicrob Ag Chemother 1989; 33: 742
4 Drugs 1990; 39: 597
5 Cancer Res 1989; 49: 2415
6 Antimicrob Ag Chemother 1980; 18: 709
7 Proc Nat Acad Sci USA 1985; 82: 7096
8 Clin Pharmacokinet 1983; 8: 187
9 J Clin Pharmac 1977; 17: 704
10 Lancet 1985; 2: 648
11 New Engl J Med 1986; 314: 801
12 Prescr J 1981; 21: 159
13 Clin Pharmac Ther 1980; 27: 690
14 New Engl J Med 1987; 316: 557

Pharmacokinetic data on anxiolytic and hypnotic agents

	pKa	logP	Oral abs %	Bio %	Tmax h	Vd l/kg	PrBd %	Met	T½ h	CL ml/min	AU %	Ref
Alprazolam	2.4	3.2C	>90		1-2	1	70	+	6-20	70	20	1
Bromazepam	*2.8	1.7	good		1-4	1	40-70		8-19	40	<5	2
Brotizolam	2.8			70		0.7	90		4-8	120	<1	3
Chloral hydrate	10.0	0.6		low		0.6		+	0.06		<1	4
Chlordiazepoxide	4.6	2.4	c100	c100	2-6	0.3-0.6	90-97	+	5-30	15-35	<1	5
Chlormethiazole	3.2		good		0.6	3-12	60-70		3-7	700-1700	<5	6
Chlormezanone		1.6C	good		4		50		20-30		<5	7
Clobazam		1.0	>90	87	1	1-2	85-90	+	10-60	35		8
Clonazepam	*1.5	2.4	good	>80	1-4	2-4	85		24-48	70-100	<1	9
Clorazepate	*3.5	2.3C				**1-3	**>95	+	**2	***7-21		10
Diazepam	3.3	2.8	100	75	1-2	0.5-2.5	>98	+	20-95	20-35	<1	11
Flunitrazepam	1.8	2.1	100	80-90	1-2	3.7	77-80	+	19-36	260	<5	12
Flurazepam	*1.9	4.5C	good		1	3.4	>95	+	2		<1	13
Hydroxyzine	*7.1	4.2C			2-4			+	3			14
Ketazolam		3.7C	good					+	1.5		<1	15
Loratidine		5.2						+	8-11			16
Lorazepam	*1.3	2.5	good	c95	1-2	1-2	90		9-24	70	<1	17

Continued on next page

Pharmacokinetic data on anxiolytic and hypnotic agents

	pKa	logP	Oral abs %	Bio %	Tmax h	Vd l/kg	PrBd %	Met	T½ h	CL ml/min	AU %	Ref
Medazepam	6.2	4.4	good		1		>95	+	1-2			18
Meprobamate		0.7	good		3.5		20		6-17	50	10-20	19
Methaqualone	2.5	2.5	good		2-3	0.7	high		10-40		<5	20
Midazolam	6.1	3.7C	iv			1.2-2	95	+	3	700-1700	<1	21
Molindone	6.9	2.6C	good		1-2						<5	22
Nitrazepam	*3.4	2.3	good		1-2	2.5	85		30	60	<10	23
Oxazepam	*1.7	2.2	good		1-4	0.5-2	95		4-25	70-140	<5	24
Prazepam	2.7	3.7	var		2-8	**0.5-3		+	**70	**5-20	<1	25
Quazepam		4.0	good		1.5			+	39			26
Temazepam	*1.3	2.2	50-85		2	1	>95	+	15-20	65	<1	27
Triazolam		3.2C	c100		1	1	80		3	330		28
Trichloroethanol***					2-9		35		7-10			29
Zopiclone	1.0C		good	c80	<1	0.6	45		2-3		<5	30

* = more than one ionizable group ; ** data for active metabolite
*** metabolite of chloral hydrate

Clinical data on anxiolytic and hypnotic agents

	Dose mg/day	Ther conc mg/l	CSF/Pl	Milk/Pl	T½ RF	T½ HF	Preg Risk Trim	Drug Int	Ref
								As a class:	
Alprazolam	0.75-1.5	0.01-0.02			0	+	3	alcohol	31
Bromazepam	3-18	0.1-0.2					3	cns depressants	32
Brotizolam							3	antiepileptics	33
Chloral hydrate	500-2000	hydrolyses					C/I		34
Chlordiazepoxide	30-100	0.4-4.0			+	+	3		35
Chlormethiazole	200-400	0.1-2.8				+			36
Chlormezanone	600-800	2.5-3.4					3		37
Clobazam	20-30	0.3-0.5					3		38
Clonazepam		0.01			0		3		39
Clorazepate	7.5-22.5	0.15-0.2					3		40
Diazepam	15-30	0.1-2.5	yes	0.16	0	+	3		41
Flunitrazepam	1-2	0.01		low		0			42
Flurazepam	15-30	0.06 met			0				43
Hydroxyzine	200-400	0.07-0.09					C/I		44
Ketazolam	15-60	c 0.004					3		45

Continued on next page

Clinical data on anxiolytic and hypnotic agents (Continued)

	Dose mg/day	Ther conc mg/l	CSF/Pl	Milk/Pl	T½ RF	T½ HF	Preg Risk Trim	Drug Int	Ref
Loratidine	5-10	0.003		low	0	0			46
Lorazepam	1-4	0.05-0.25	<1		+	+	3	alcohol	47
Medazepam	15-30	0.14-0.26					3		48
Meprobamate	1200-1600	5-20			+		3	oral contraceptives	49
Methaqualone	150-300			avoid	+				50
Midazolam	2.5-7.5 iv				0	+	3		51
Molindone	50-100								52
Nitrazepam	5-10	0.08-0.1	0.2				3		53
Oxazepam	45-120	0.5-2.0			+	0	3		54
Prazepam	10-60	0.2-0.4					3		55
Quazepam	10-25	0.1		4.0					56
Temazepam	20-40	0.9	0.05				3		57
Triazolam	0.13-0.25				0		3		58
Trichloroethanol									59
Zopiclone	5-10			avoid		+		cns depressants	60

72

References

1 Clin Therap 1991; 13: 100
2 J Pharmacokinet Biopharm 1976;
  4: 1
3 Br J Clin Pharmac 1983; 16:
  Suppl 2, 200S
4 Clin Pharmac Ther 1973; 14: 147
5 Clin Pharmacokinet 1978; 3: 381
6 Eur J Clin Pharmac 1977; 12: 137
7 Anzneim Forsch 1986; 36: 1116
8 Drugs 1980; 20: 161
9 Analyt Prof Drug Subs 1977; 6:
  61
10 Eur J Clin Pharmac 1985; 28:
   229
11 Clin Pharmacokinet 1978; 3: 72
12 Clin Pharmacokinet 1986; 11: 18
13 Clin Pharmacokinet 1976; 1: 426
14 J Pharm Sci 1979; 68: 1456
15 Clin Pharmacokinet 1983; 8: 233
16 J Clin Pharmac 1987; 27: 530
17 Clin Pharmacokinet 1981; 6: 89
18 Br J Clin Pharmac 1977; 4: 51
19 Chemotherapie 1964; 9: 20
20 J Pharmacokinet Biopharm 1978;
   6: 111
21 Clin Pharmacokinet 1986; 11: 18
22 Clin Ther 1985; 7: 169
23 Br J Clin Pharmac 1977; 4: 709
24 Clin Pharmacokinet 1981; 6: 89
25 J Clin Pharmac 1984; 24: 446
26 Drug Met Dispos 1985; 13: 25
27 Biopharm Drug Disposit 1990;
   11: 499
28 Clin Pharmacokinet 1983; 8: 233
29 Clin Pharmac Ther 1973; 14: 147
30 Int J Clin Pharmac Ther Tox
   1985; 23: 97
31 Hosp Formulary 1991; 26: Suppl
   A, 2
32 J Pharm Sci 1973; 62: 1776
33 Br J Clin Pharmac 1983; 16:
   285S
34 Clin Pharmac Ther 1977; 21: 355
35 Eur J Clin Pharmac 1978; 13:
   267
36 Eur J Clin Pharmac 1980; 17:
   275
37 Eur J Drug Met Pharmacokinet
   1991; 16: 43
38 Br J Clin Pharmac 1987; 23: 137
39 Psychosomatics 1985; 26: Suppl
   7
40 Eur J Clin Pharmac 1979; 15:
   171
41 New Engl J Med 1983; 309: 354
42 Fundam Clin Pharmac 1990; 4:
   643
43 Clin Pharmac Ther 1977; 21: 355
44 Curr Ther Res 1984; 35: 715
45 Drug Ther Bull 1980; 18: 94
46 Drugs 1989; 37: 42
47 Clin Pharmac Ther 1977; 21: 222
48 Br J Anaesth 1975; 47: 464
49 Drugs 1979; 17: 198
50 Br J Clin Pharmac 1982; 14: 333
51 Gut 1986; 27: 190
52 J Clin Pharmac 1981; 21: 351
53 Clin Pharmac Ther 1985; 38: 697
54 Drugs 1978; 16: 358
55 J Clin Pharmac 1984; 24: 446
56 Pharmacotherapy 1990; 10: 1
57 Eur J Clin Pharmac 1990; 38:
   153
58 Drugs 1981; 22: 81
59 Clin Pharmac Ther 1972; 13: 37
60 Int J Psychopharmac 1990; 5: 147

Pharmacokinetic data on barbiturates and related agents

	pKa	logP	Oral abs %	Bio %	Tmax h	Vd l/kg	PrBd %	Met	T½ h	CL ml/min	AU %	Ref
Amylobarbitone	7.9	1.6	c100	95	1-3	1	40-60	+	8-40	35	1	1
Butobarbitone	8.0	1.7	good		1-2	0.8	26		34-42	15	5-9	2
Cyclobarbitone	7.6	1.8	good		1-3	0.5	70		8-17	35	<10	3
Methyprylone	12.0	0.8			2			+	4		3	4
Pentobarbitone	8.0	2.1	good		1-2		50		35-50			5
Phenobarbitone	7.4	1.4	c100	>90	0.5-4	0.5-0.7	50		c100	5	25	6
Quinalbarbitone	7.9	2.0	90		3	1.5	50-70		19-34	56	10-20	7
Secbutobarbitone											5-9	8

Clinical data on barbiturates and related agents

	Dose mg/day	Ther conc mg/l	CSF/Pl	Milk/Pl	T½ RF	T½ HF	Preg Risk Trim	Drug Int	Ref
								As a class:	
Amylobarbitone	100-200	2-12	+				C/I	alcohol	9
Butobarbitone	100-200	2-15				+	C/I	cns depressants	10
Cyclobarbitone	100-400	2-10					C/I	phenytoin	11
Methyprylone	200-400	10-20							12
Pentobarbitone	100-200	1-4			0	+			13
Phenobarbitone	60-180	2-30		avoid	+		C/I	anticoagulants	14
Quinalbarbitone	50-100	2-10	+		0		C/I		15
Secbutobarbitone	50-100								16

References

1 Clin Pharmacokinet 1977; 2: 93
2 Eur J Clin Pharmac 1976; 10: 263
3 Eur J Clin Pharmac 1976; 9: 440
4 Arch Int Pharmacodyn Ther 1956; 106: 388
5 Drug Intell Clin Pharm 1987; 21: 459
6 Analyt Prof Drug Subs 1978; 7: 359
7 Clin Pharmac Ther 1974; 16: 376
8 J Pharm Pharmac 1975; 27: 923
9 Br J Clin Pharmac 1974; 1: 41
10 Br Med J 1983; 286: 1980
11 J Pharm Sci 1975; 64: 1576
12 J Pharm Sci 1985; 74: 1001
13 Digestion 1973; 8: 448
14 Drug Ther Bull 1987; 25: 9
15 Ann Inter Med 1980; 93: 286
16 Martindale 1989; 29th ed, 766

Pharmacokinetic data on beta-adrenoceptor antagonists

	pKa	logP	Oral abs %	Bio %	Tmax h	Vd l/kg	PrBd %	Met	T½ h	CL ml/min	AU %	Ref
Acebutolol	9.4	-0.4	90	40	2-4	1.2	20	+	3-6	500	10-55	1
Alprenolol	9.6	1.0	90	9	1	1-3	76-85	+	2-3**	117-450	5	2
Atenolol	9.6	-1.5	50	50	2-3	1.1	<5		5-9	100-180	40-50	3
Betaxolol		2.2C	100	88	1-4	6	50	+	15	320	16	4
Bevantolol	8.1	2.6C	100	60		1.5	95		2		<10	5
Bisoprolol		1.7C				3	30		10	250		6
Bopindolol		4.9C		70	1-2			+	6*			7
Bufuralol		2.7	100	55	1-3	1.8	90	+	2-4**	700	<1	8
Carteolol		-0.5	100	>95	1-2		16	+	5-7		70-90	9
Celiprolol	9.7	1.7C	80	55	2-4	2-3	26		4-6	130-180	11-28	10
Dilevalol	9.5	1.2		30	2	17			12	2100		11
Epanolol		1.0C		8	1-2	4	50		19	2000	<2	12
Esmolol	9.5	1.5C	iv			3	55		0.2	230000	<2	13

Continued on next page

Pharmacokinetic data on beta-adrenoceptor antagonists (Continued)

	pKa	logP	Oral abs %	Bio %	Tmax h	Vd l/kg	PrBd %	Met	T½ h	CL ml/min	AU %	Ref
Labetalol	8.7	1.2	90	30	1	10	50		2-6	1500	<5	14
Levobunolol	9.3	2.3C	good	75	1-3	5		+	6	800	15	15
Metoprolol	9.7	-0.1	>95	50	1-2	6	12	+	2-5**	1000	<5	16
Nadolol	9.7	-1.3	25	25	2-5	2	20-30		15	150	25	17
Nipradilol		1.9C										18
Oxprenolol	9.5	0.3	90	50	1-2	1.2	80-95		2-3	200	<5	19
Pafenolol		1.7C	iv			1.1			3-4**	300	50	20
Penbutolol	9.3	1.9	>95	50	1-2	1	98	+	5-27		<5	21
Pindolol	8.8	0.0	>95	90	1-3		60		3-4	530	40	22
Practolol	9.5	-1.7	>95	95	1-3		7		10	140	85	23
Propranolol	9.5	1.3	100	35	1-4	3	85-95	+	3-4	1000	<5	24
Sotalol	9.8	-1.3	100	100	2-3	1	<5		15	150	60-75	25
Timolol	8.8	-0.1	72	60	1-2	2	60		3-6**	500	20	26

* for active metabolite   ** = genetic polymorphism

Clinical data on beta-adrenoceptor antagonists

	Dose mg/day	Ther conc mg/l	CSF/Pl	Milk/Pl	T½ RF	T½ HF	Preg Risk Trim	Drug Int	Ref
Acebutolol	400	0.2-2	low	>1	+	0	3	As a class:	27
Alprenolol	100	0.05-0.1	high	>1	0	+	3	verapamil	28
Atenolol	50-100	0.2-0.6	low	avoid	+	0	3	clondidine	29
Betaxolol	20-40	0.005-0.02			0	0	3	hypoglycaemics	30
Bevantolol	200-400				+	0	3	sympathomimetics	31
Bisoprolol									32
Bopindolol	1-2	0.006				+			33
Bufuralol	30-60	0.01-0.1					3	reserpine	34
Carteolol	15-30	0.005-0.01					3	other antihypertensives	35
Celiprolol	600	0.05-0.4			+	0	3	cimetidine	36
Dilevalol	400	0.02							37
Epanolol	200	0.02-0.04			+	0	3	ergot alkaloids	38
Esmolol	0.3/kg/min	2						cns depressants	39

Continued on next page

Clinical data on beta-adrenoceptor antagonists (Continued)

	Dose mg/day	Ther conc mg/l	CSF/Pl	Milk/Pl	T½ RF	T½ HF	Preg Risk Trim	Drug Int	Ref
Labetalol	200-400	0.05-0.1	low	<1	0	+	3	indomethacin	40
Levobunolol	2% eye	0.2-0.3							41
Metoprolol	100-400	0.05-0.1	high	3-4	0	0	3		42
Nadolol	80-240	0.04-0.1	low	4,avoid	+	0	3		43
Nipradilol									44
Oxprenolol	80-480	0.04-0.1	high	<1	0		3		45
Pafenolol									46
Penbutolol	40-80	0.05-0.2					3		47
Pindolol	15-45	0.05-0.15	fair		+	0	3		48
Practolol	5 iv	1.5-5	fair		+		3		49
Propranolol	160-320	0.05-0.1	high	0.3-0.8	0	+	3		50
Sotalol	160-600	0.5-4	0.1	caution	+	0	3		51
Timolol	10-60	0.005-0.01			0		3		52

80

References

1 Drugs 1985; 29: 531
2 Clin Pharmac Ther 1977; 22: 545
3 Drugs 1983; 25: Suppl 2
4 Eur J Clin Pharmac 1986; 31: 231
5 Drugs 1988; 35: 1
6 J Chromatogr 1987; 403: 263
7 Drugs 1991; 41: 130
8 Eur J Clin Pharmac 1985; 28: 317
9 Eur J Clin Pharmac 1983; 25: 95
10 Drugs 1987; 34: 438
11 Clin Pharmac Ther 1989; 46: 648
12 Drugs 1989; 38: Suppl 2, 10
13 J Clin Pharmac 1986; 26: 44
14 Clin Pharmacokinet 1984; 9: 157
15 Drugs 1987; 34: 648
16 Br J Clin Pharmac 1981; 11: 287
17 J Clin Pharmac 1979; 19: 712
18 Clin Pharm Bull 1985; 33: 3456
19 Clin Pharmac Ther 1976; 20: 401
20 Biopharm Drug Disposit 1990;
   11: 607
21 J Clin Pharmac 1977; 17: 231
22 Eur J Clin Pharmac 1983; 25:
   357
23 Clin Pharmac Ther 1973; 14: 26
24 Clin Pharmac Ther 1986; 40: 29
25 Drugs 1987; 34: 311
26 Clin Pharmac Ther 1985; 38: 409
27 Br Med J 1983; 286: 1043
28 Clin Pharmac Ther 1977; 22: 316
29 Drugs 1990; 40: 75
30 Eur J Clin Pharmac 1990; 38:
   477
31 Drugs 1988; 35: 1
32 Br J Clin Pharmac 1987; 23:
   623P
33 Eur J Clin Pharmac 1990; 39:
   569
34 Int J Clin Pharmac Biopharm
   1978; 16: 54
35 Clin Pharmac Ther 1984; 35: 301
36 J Card Pharmac 1986; Suppl 4,
   S75
37 J Clin Pharmac 1988; 28: 644
38 Drugs 1989; 38: Suppl 2, 18
39 Drugs 1987; 33: 392
40 Br J Clin Pharmac 1982; 13:
   Suppl 1
41 Am J Opthalm 1985; 99: 18
42 Pharm Res 1990; 7: 953
43 Br J Clin Pharmac 1985; 19: 37
44 Arch Int Pharmacodyn 1983;
   262: 132
45 Eur J Clin Pharmac 1975; 8: 3
46 J Chromatogr 1982; 242: 41
47 Br J Clin Pharmac 1977; 4: 135
48 New Engl J Med 1983; 308: 940
49 Br Med J 1973; 2: 177
50 Clin Pharmac Ther 1983; 34: 440
51 Br J Clin Pharmac 1990; 29: 277
52 Br Med J 1982; 285: 84

Pharmacokinetic data on calcium antagonists and peripheral vasodilators

	pKa	logP	Oral abs %	Bio %	Tmax h	Vd l/kg	PrBd %	Met	T½ h	CL ml/min	AU %	Ref
Amlodipine	*9,0	2.8C		52-88		21	97		30-40	450		1
Bamethan		1.5C			0.5-1						30	2
Cinnarizine		6.1C			2							3
Diltiazem	7.7	2.7	c100	40	3	4.5	>95		3-5	1000	<5	4
Felodipine	**	7.1	c100	15	0.5-2	4-10	>99		25	800	<1	5
Gallopamil		3.1C	c100	15					3-6			6
Isradipine	**	4.3	c100	17	1	69-161	>90		9-16	750	<5	7
Lidoflazine		5.8	high		1				24			8
Nicardipine	**	4.3C	c100	35	0.3-2	0.8	>90		7-12	580	<5	9
Nifedipine	**	3.3	c100	50	1-2	1-1.5	>90		2-4	100-700	<1	10
Nilvadipine		2.1C		14			98		11	1250	<1	11
Nimodipine	**	6.0	c100	5-13	1-2	1-2.5	>95		1-13	1000-13000	<10	12
Nisoldipine	**	7.1	c100	4-8	1-2	2-3	>90		2-3	1250	<5	13
Nitrendipine	**	6.0	c 80	low	1-2	5-6	>99		5-7	1300	<5	14
Oxypentifylline	0.3		high	low	1-1.5	5		+	0.4-1	4900	<1	15
Prenylamine		5.5C	high				>95	+	7			16
Thymoxamine			poor		0.5-1							17
Tiapamil		0.6C		15-70		2	78		2-3	670-750		18
Verapamil	8.9	3.8	c100	20	2-3	4-5	90	+	2-7	700-1400	<5	19

* = more than one ionizable group ; ** = very weak bases

Pharmacokinetic data on calcium antagonists and peripheral vasodilators

	Dose mg/day	Ther conc mg/l	CSF/Pl	Milk/Pl	TV RF	TV HF	Preg Risk Trim	Drug Int	Ref
Amlodipine	10-15								20
Bamethan	100	0.04-0.12							21
Cinnarizine	225	0.08						cns depressants	22
Diltiazem	180-360			cl,avoid	0		S/P	digitalis	23
Felodipine	10-20	0.002-0.01					C/I	anticonvulsants	24
Gallopamil	100								25
Isradipine	2.5-10				+	+		anticonvulsants	26
Lidoflazine	120-360	0.12					3	beta-blockers	27
Nicardipine	30-90						C/I	digoxin	28
Nifedipine	10-60			cl	0	+	C/I	quinidine	29
Nilvadipine	2-6								30
Nimodipine	90-120	0.05	low		+	+			31
Nisoldipine	30-60				0	+		cimetidine	32
Nitrendipine	40			0.5-1.4	0	+			33
Oxypentifylline	800-1200	1.5						antihypertensives	34
Prenylamine									35
Thymoxamine	160	0.06						tricyclics	36
Tiapamil	600					+		digoxin	37
Verapamil	120-480	0.26		0.6		+	3	quinidine	38

References

1 Br J Clin Pharmac 1986; 22: 21
2 Arzneim Forsch 1981; 31: 843
3 Drugs 1983; 26: 44
4 Eur J Drug Met Pharmacokinet 1991; 16: 75
5 Drugs 1987; 34: Suppl 3
6 Z Kardiol 1989; 78: Suppl 15, 20
7 Eur J Clin Pharmac 1987; 32: 361
8 Br Med J 1981; 282: 400
9 Postgrad Med J 1984; 60: Suppl 4
10 Drugs 1985; 30: 182
11 J Clin Pharmac 1987; 27: 293
12 Pharmac Res 1987; 4: Suppl 2
13 Drugs 1987; 34: 578
14 Drugs 1987; 33: 123
15 Drugs 1987; 34: 50
16 Arzneim Forsch 1973; 23: 74
17 J Pharm Pharmac 1971; 23: 719
18 Eur J Clin Pharmac 1986; 31: 397
19 Clin Pharmacokinet 1984; 9: 26
20 Clin Pharmacokinet 1988; 15: 1
21 Arzneim Forsch 1968; 18: 1212
22 Drug Ther Bull 1981; 19: 27
23 Eur J Clin Pharmac 1983; 24: 635
24 Drugs of Today 1989; 25: 589
25 Am J Cardiol 1984; 53: 684
26 Clin Pharmac Ther 1990; 48: 590
27 Drug Ther Bull 1983; 21: 27
28 J Am Coll Cardiol 1984; 4: 908
29 New Engl J Med 1982; 307: 1618
30 Cardiov Drug Rev 1988; 6: 97
31 Drugs 1989; 37: 669
32 J Am Coll Cardiol 1985; 6: 447
33 Eur J Clin Pharmac 1985; 28: 473
34 Drugs 1987; 34: 50
35 Arzneim Forsch 1973; 23: 74
36 Curr Med Res Opin 1982; 8: 158
37 Clin Ther 1983; 5: 595
38 New Engl J Med 1985; 313: 995

Pharmacokinetic data on cardiovascular agents

	pKa	logP	Oral abs %	Bio %	Tmax h	Vd l/kg	PrBd %	Met	T½ h	CL ml/min	AU %	Ref
Cardiac glycosides												
Digitoxin		1.8	good	>90	2-3	0.4-0.8	95	+	c 200	3	20-50	1
Digoxin		1.3	var	c 70	1	5-10	20-40	+	20-50	70-240	60-80	2
Lanatoside C		0.1	poor		1	4	25	+	40		c 70	3
Medigoxin			>90		1	6-10	10-30	+	40-70	140	30-50	4
Ouabain	6.0C		var				10-40		10-20		40-50	5
Diuretics												
Amiloride	8.7		<90	50		5	low		6-10	500	50	6
Bendrofluazide	8.5		>90		2-3	1-2	95		4-9	250	30	7
Bumetanide		4.1C	100		1-8	0.2	95		1-2	210	30-50	8
Chlorothiazide	* 9.5	-2.0	poor	<30	1		95		2-13			9
Chlorthalidone	9.4	0.2C	<90	65	1-3	4	75		35-70	70-140	25-50	10
Ethacrynic acid	3.5	3.2C	good						0.5-1		20	11
Frusemide	3.9	2.3C	<90	65	1	0.1-0.2	95		1-3	70-210	70-90	12
Hydrochlorothiazide	* 9.2	-0.1	<90	70	2-4	3	40		6-15	350	65-70	13

Continued on next page

Pharmacokinetic data on cardiovascular agents (Continued)

	pKa	logP	Oral abs %	Bio %	Tmax h	Vd l/kg	PrBd %	Met	T½ h	CL ml/min	AU %	Ref
Hydroflumethiazide	*10	0.4	<90		2-4		75-95		5-18		50-70	14
Indapamide	8.3		100		2-3		80		15	20	5-10	15
Mefruside		1.4C	c 90			6			3-12	350-210C	<1	16
Metolazone	9.7	2.6C	40-65		5	1-2	95		18	100	70-80	17
Piretanide		3.9C	c100		1	0.3	>90		1-2	200	51	18
Polythiazide	9.8	2.5C	good		5-12		80-85		25		20	19
Spironolactone		2.3C	<90		2-3		**>95	+	**18		low	20
Torasemide			80		1	0.1-0.3			1-6	70	22-34	21
Triamterene	6.2	1.1	<90	50	1-2		45-70	+	2-4	1600	5-10	22
Xipamide	*10	1.5C	100		1		>95		5-8	19	30-50	23

* = more than one ionizable group ; ** active metabolite

Clinical data on cardiovascular agents

	Dose mg/day	Ther conc mg/l	CSF/Pl	Milk/Pl	T½ RF	T½ HF	Preg Risk Trim	Drug Int	Ref
Cardiac glycosides									
Digitoxin	0.05-0.2	0.01-0.03			+			glycosides	24
Digoxin	1-1.5	0.001-0.002		0.6-0.9	+			quinidine	25
Lanatoside C	1.5-2	0.0005-0.001							26
Medigoxin	0.4	0.0006-0.002							27
Ouabain	1 iv	0.0005			+				28
Diuretics									
Amiloride	10-20				avoid		3	ace inhibitors	29
Bendrofluazide	5-10	0.07-0.1					3	digitalis	30
Bumetanide	1-2	0.03					3	lithium	31
Chlorothiazide	500-2000	0.5-1.4					3	antihypertensives	32
Chlorthalidone	25-50	0.2-1.4			+		3		33
Ethacrynic acid	50-150				avoid		3	warfarin	34
Frusemide	20-80	1.8-5.0			+		3	nsaids	35
Hydrochlorothiazide	25-200	0.05-0.15			avoid	+	3		36

Continued on next page

Clinical data on cardiovascular agents (Continued)

	Dose mg/day	Ther conc mg/l	CSF/Pl	Milk/Pl	T½ RF	T½ HF	Preg Risk Trim	Drug Int	Ref
Hydroflumethiazide	25-50	0.17-0.6					3		37
Indapamide	2.5	0.02-0.05					3		38
Mefruside	25-50	0.07-0.13					3		39
Metolazone	2.5-10	0.01					3		40
Piretanide	6-12						3		41
Polythiazide	1-4	0.002-0.007					3		42
Spironolactone	100-400	0.2			avoid		3		43
Torasemide	10-20								44
Triamterene	150-300	0.13-0.15			avoid		3	K supplements	45
Xipamide	20-40	5				0	3		46

References

1 Clin Pharmacokinet 1985; 10: 514
2 Clin Pharmacokinet 1980; 5: 137
3 Clin Pharmac Ther 1977; 21: 647
4 Eur J Clin Pharmac 1977; 12: 387
5 New Engl J Med 1973; 289: 1063
6 Clin Pharmac Ther 1969; 10: 401
7 Clin Pharmac Ther 1977; 22: 385
8 Clin Pharmacokinet 1987; 12: 440
9 Pharm J 1981; 2: 265
10 Eur J Clin Pharmac 1980; 17: 203
11 Drugs 1985; 29: 57
12 Clin Pharmacokinet 1979; 4: 279
13 Clin Pharmacokinet 1979; 4: 63
14 Eur J Clin Pharmac 1979; 16: 125
15 Clin Pharmacokinet 1987; 13: 254
16 Eur J Clin Pharmac 1980; 17: 59
17 Clin Pharmac Ther 1974; 16: 322
18 Clin Pharmacokinet 1987; 13: 254
19 Clin Pharmac Ther 1978; 23: 241
20 Drug Met Rev 1978; 8: 151
21 Drug Research 1988; 38: 164
22 Eur J Clin Pharmac 1979; 16: 39
23 Arzneim Forsch 1977; 27: 2143
24 New Engl J Med 1973; 289: 1063
25 Clin Pharmacokinet 1985; 10: 1
26 Pharm J 1982; 1: 51
27 Clin Pharmac Ther 1977; 22: 280
28 Toxicol Appl Pharmac 1971; 20: 44
29 Med Lett 1981; 23: 109
30 Br J Clin Pract 1987; 41: 967
31 Drugs 1984; 28: 426
32 Br Med J 1983; 286: 1535
33 Pharmacotherapeutica 1983; 3: 475
34 Am J Kid Dis 1983; 3: 155
35 Drugs 1985; 29: 57
36 Lancet 1984; 1: 496
37 J Clin Pharmac 1978; 18: 190
38 Drugs 1984; 28: 189
39 Arzneim Forsch 1967; 17: 653
40 J Clin Pharmac 1985; 25: 369
41 Drugs 1985; 29: 489
42 Clin Pharmac Ther 1977; 21: 105
43 Am Heart J 1978; 96: 389
44 Drugs 1991; 41: Suppl 3, 14
45 Eur J Clin Pharmac 1983; 24: 453
46 Clin Pharmac Ther 1990; 48: 628

Pharmacokinetic data on cephalosporins and other anti-infective agents

	pKa	logP	Oral abs %	Bio %	Tmax h	Vd l/kg	PrBd %	Met	T½ h	CL ml/min	AU %	Ref
Cefaclor		-2.7	90-95	90	1-2	0.3-0.5	25		0.6	500	90-95	1
Cefadroxil		-2.7	85		1-3	0.2-0.4	20		1-2	200-300	70-90	2
Cefapirin			poor			0.2	50		0.5-1	370	70	3
Cefathiamidine									0.5		90	4
Cefatrizine		-0.3C	40			0.33	60		1.4	230	75	5
Cefazaflur		-1.5C				0.35	65		0.4		90	6
Cefazedone						0.13	95		1-2		80	7
Cefbuperazone									1.6		75	8
Cefiximine		0.2C		40	3-5	0.2	70		3-4	150-320		9
Cefmenoxime					1		77		1			10
Cefmetazole		-0.6	im		0.7	0.13	85		1	90-165	75	11
Cefonicid		-1.7C	im		1-2	0.13	98		4.4	27	95	12
Cefoperazone		-0.7	im		1-2	0.19	90		2	80	30	13
Ceforanide		-1.7C	im		1	0.2	45-85		3	40-50	85	14
Cefotaxime		-0.2C				0.4	30-40	+	1-1.5	250	50-60	15
Cefotetan		-1.2C	im		2-3	0.13	90		3.5	35	80	16
Cefotiam		-4.0C				0.36	40		0.8	390	70	17
Cefoxitin	3.5	-0.0C	im			0.2	75		1-2	250-330	77-90	18
Cefpimizole						0.27			2	119	80	19
Cefpiramide		0.5C				0.1	96		5		25	20
Cefpodoxime		0.6C		50		0.3			2-3	200	40	21

Continued on next page

Pharmacokinetic data on cephalosporins and other anti-infective agents (Continued)

	pKa	logP	Oral abs %	Bio %	Tmax h	Vd l/kg	PrBd %	Met	T½ h	CL ml/min	AU %	Ref
Cefroxadine		-0.2C	90			0.2	10	+	1	340	80-96	22
Cefsulodin			85			0.2-0.4	30		1.5	80-145	60-70	23
Cefsumide		-1.0C	90				13		2-4		90	24
Ceftazidime						0.2-0.3	15		2	110	60-90	25
Ceftezole		-2.2C	3				85		0.9-3		90	26
Ceftizoxime						0.2-0.3	30		1.7	130-160	70-100	27
Ceftriaxone	* 3.2					0.1-0.2	83-96		8.5	20	65	28
Cefuroxime	2.5	-0.2	low			0.2-0.3	40		1.3	130	>90	29
Cephacetrile		-0.5	95			0.27	25		0.7		75	30
Cephalexin	* 2.5	0.7	90		1-2	0.2-0.3	10-15		0.8-1	250-380	50-90	31
Cephaloglycin	* 4.6	-1.3C	25				25		1-2		15	32
Cephaloridine	3.4					0.21	20		1.4	170	70	33
Cephalothin	2.2	0.5				0.2-0.3	65-70		0.5	330-470	60-90	34
Cephamandole		0.5				0.2	75		0.8	220-260	80-100	35
Cephazolin	2.1	-0.2	low			0.13	80-85		1.8-2	50-65	65-95	36
Cephradine	* 2.5	-1.2	95			0.25	10		0.8	280-580	100	37
Latamoxef						0.2	50		2.5	70-115	75	38
Others												
Aztreonam	* 2.8	-1.6C	iv,im			0.2	55-60		1.5-2	100	75	39
Clavulanic acid					1	0.2	27		1	220	30-40	40
Clioquinol	* 8.1	3.4C	var		4				11-14		<1	41
Iodoquinol	* 8.0	4.0C	var									42

* = more than one ionizable group

Clinical data on cephalosporins and other anti-infective agents

	Dose mg/day	Ther conc mg/l	CSF/Pl	Milk/Pl	T½ RF	T½ HF	Preg Risk Trim	Drug Int	Ref
Cefaclor	1000-4000	10-15						As a class:	43
Cefadroxil	1000-2000			<0.05	+			loop diuretics	44
Cefapirin	1000 im	16-24		low	+				45
Cefathiamidine									46
Cefatrizine									47
Cefazaflur	1000 im	25							48
Cefazedone	6000 im								49
Cefbuperazone	1000 iv								50
Cefixime	400	1-2			+				51
Cefmenoxime	1000-4000 im				+				52
Cefmetazole	30 mg/kg im	90			+				53
Cefonicid	1000 im	67-126							54
Cefoperazone	1000-2000 im	65-97		low					55
Ceforanide	500-1000 im	38-70			+	+			56
Cefotaxime	<12000 im	12-25	*+	<0.05	+			aminoglycosides	57
Cefotetan	1000-2000 im	65-90		low					58
Cefotiam									59
Cefoxitin	<12000 im	30	low	<0.05	+				60
Cefpimizole									61
Cefpiramide									62
Cefpodoxime	100-800	1-3							63

Continued on next page

Clinical data on cephalosporins and other anti-infective agents (Continued)

	Dose mg/day	Ther conc mg/l	CSF/Pl	Milk/Pl	T½ RF	T½ HF	Preg Risk Trim	Drug Int	Ref
Cefroxadine	1000 iv	10							64
Cefsulodin	1000-4000 im				+				65
Cefsumide									66
Ceftazidime	3000-4000 im		* +		+				67
Ceftezole									68
Ceftizoxime	1000-8000 im	40-160	0.2	<0.05	+				69
Ceftriaxone	1000-3000 im		* +		+				70
Cefuroxime									71
Cephacetrile		3							72
Cephalexin	1000-2000	6-50		<0.05	+				73
Cephaloglycin									74
Cephaloridine		0.1-15							75
Cephalothin	<12000 iv				+				76
Cephamandole	<12000 iv	0.5-5	* +		+				77
Cephazolin	<4000 im,iv	0.1-50			+				78
Cephradine	1000-4000	0.5-10	* +	0.2	+				79
Latamoxef									80
Others									
Aztreonam	<4000 im,iv	5-10	+	<0.01	+	+	C/I		81
Clavulanic acid		2-3							82
Clioquinol	topical	0.3-1.3							83
Iodoquinol									84

* = penetration in meningitis

References

1 Analyt Prof Drug Subs 1980; 9: 107
2 Drugs 1986; 32: Suppl 3, 1
3 J Pharm Sci 1975; 64: 1899
4 Antimicrob Ag Chemother 1972; 1: 54
5 Antimicrob Ag Chemother 1976; 9: 800
6 J Clin Pharmac 1977; 17: 128
7 Arzneim Forsch 1979; 29: 361
8 Chemotherapy (Tokyo) 1982; 30: 212
9 Clin Pharmac Ther 1985; 38: 590
10 Antimicrob Ag Chemother 1982; 21: 141
11 Antimicrob Ag Chemother 1985; 28: 544
12 Drugs 1986; 32: 222
13 Antimicrob Ag Chemother 1981; 19: 298
14 Antimicrob Ag Chemother 1982; 21: 323
15 J Pharmacokinet Biopharm 1985; 13: 121
16 Drugs 1985; 30: 382
17 Antimicrob Ag Chemother 1982; 22: 958
18 Analyt Prof Drug Subs 1982; 11: 195
19 Antimicrob Ag Chemother 1980; 26: 802
20 Antimicrob Ag Chemother 1984; 25: 221
21 J Antimicrob Chemother 1990; 26: Suppl E, 21
22 J Pharmacokinet Biopharm 1982; 10: 15
23 Antimicrob Ag Chemother 1984; 25: 579
24 J Antibiot 1976; 29: 444
25 Antimicrob Ag Chemother 1990; 34: 2307
26 Antimicrob Ag Chemother 1976; 10: 1
27 Drugs 1985; 29: 281
28 Drugs 1984; 27: 469
29 J Antimicrob Chemother 1979; 5: 183
30 J Pharm Sci 1975; 64: 1899
31 Postgrad Med J 1983; 59: Suppl 5, 16
32 J Pharm Sci 1975; 64: 1899
33 J Pharm Sci 1975; 64: 1899
34 J Pharm Sci 1975; 64: 1899
35 J Infect Dis 1978; 137: Suppl May, S80
36 Clin Pharmac Ther 1980; 27: 550
37 Clin Pharmac Ther 1975; 18: 215
38 Drugs 1983; 26: 279
39 Antimicrob Ag Chemother 1983; 24: 394
40 Antimicrob Ag Chemother 1982; 21: 681
41 J Pharm Sci 1973; 62: 1929
42 J Pharm Sci 1966; 55: 730
43 Curr Med Res Opin 1981; 7: 168
44 Drugs 1986; 32: 1
45 Chemotherapy (Basle) 1976; 22: 274
46 Chin Med J 1979; 92: 26
47 Drugs 1980; 20: 137
48 Drugs of Today 1976; 12: 171
49 Arzneim Forsch 1979; 29: 361
50 Chemotherapy (Tokyo) 1982; 30: 212
51 Jpn J Antibiot 1987; 40: 1537
52 Drugs 1987; 34: 188
53 Antimicrob Ag Chemother 1990; 34: 1944
54 Drugs 1986; 32: 222

References *(continued)*

55 Drugs 1981; 22: 423
56 Drugs 1987; 34: 41157 Drugs
    1983; 25: 223
58 J Antimicrob Chemother 1983;
    11: Suppl A1
59 Int J Pharmaceut 1984; 19: 345
60 Drugs 1979; 17: 1
61 Antimicrob Ag Chemother 1987;
    31: 1706
62 Antimicrob Ag Chemother 1987;
    32: 1585
63 J Antimicrob Chemother 1990;
    26: Supp E, 41
64 Int J Clin Pharmac Ther Tox
    1990; 28: 435
65 Clin Pharmacokinet 1984; 3: 373
66 J Antibiot 1976; 29: 444
67 Med Lett 1985; 27: 85
68 Chemotherapy, Tokyo 1976; 24:
    573
69 J Antimicrob Chemother 1982;
    10: Suppl C 1

70 Med Lett 1985; 27: 37
71 Med Lett 1984; 26: 15
72 Eur J Clin Pharmac 1979; 16: 49
73 Postgrad Med J 1983; 59: Suppl
    5, 1
74 J Antibiot 1981; 34: 1641
75 Br J Opthalm 1973; 57: 421
76 Med Lett 1986; 28: 33
77 Ann Intern Med 1985; 103: 70
78 Drugs 1986; 31: 449
79 Clin Pharmacokinet 1987; 12:
    136
80 Med Lett 1982; 24: 13
81 Antimicrob Ag Chemother 1984;
    26: 493
82 Ther Drug Monit 1984; 6: 424
83 Analyt Prof Drug Subs 1989; 18:
    57
84 Clin Pharmac Ther 1968; 9: 67

Pharmacokinetic data on cerebral vasodilators and sympathomimetics

	pKa	logP	Oral abs %	Bio %	Tmax h	Vd l/kg	PrBd %	Met	T½ h	CL ml/min	AU %	Ref
Adrenaline	*8.7	-1.4	poor	0							<1	1
Dobutamine	9.5	2.2C	inact	0			50		0.05	4000		2
Dopamine	*8.8	0.4	inact	0		0.2			0.05	4000-6000		3
Isoprenaline	*8.6	0.1C	irreg		1-2	0.5			0.05		<5	4
Isoxsuprine	*8.0	2.6C	good		1		70		1.5			5
Metaraminol	8.6	-0.3						+	<0.1			6
Naftidrofuryl	8.2				0.5-1							7
Noradrenaline	*8.6	-1.1C									16	8
Phenylephrine	*8.9	-0.3	irreg	38	1-2	5			2-3	2100	<1	9
Prenalterol	*9.5	1.1C				2.4	low		2-3	800		10

* = more than one ionizable group

Clinical data on cerebral vasodilators and sympathomimetics

	Dose mg/day	Ther conc mg/l	CSF/Pl	Milk/Pl	T½ RF	T½ HF	Preg Risk Trim	Drug Int	Ref
Adrenaline	0.5 iv,im							maois	11
Dobutamine	iv infusion								12
Dopamine	iv infusion								13
Isoprenaline	240-840							anaesthetics	14
Isoxsuprine	80								15
Metaraminol	15-100 iv						C/I		16
Naftidrofuryl	400 iv								17
Noradrenaline	rapid iv						C/I		18
Phenylephrine	5 im,sc	0.001					C/I		19
Prenalterol	5-10 iv	0.05							20

References

1 J Pharm Sci 1977; 66: 447
2 Clin Pharmac Ther 1978; 24: 537
3 Am J Hosp Pharm 1979; 36: 881
4 J Pharm Pharmac 1974; 26: 265
5 J Paediatr 1981; 98: 146
6 Clin Pharmacokinet 1986; 5: 572
7 J Eur Toxicol 1969; 11: 40
8 Clin Pharmac Ther 1979; 26: 669
9 Anaesth Analg Curr Res 1973;
  52: 161
10 Biopharm Drug Disposit 1986; 7:
  47
11 New Engl J Med 1985; 312: 897
12 Ann Intern Med 1983; 99: 490
13 Br J Anaesth 1986; 58: 151
14 Prescribers J 1983; 23: 32
15 Drug Ther Bull 1980; 18: 34
16 Can Med Ass J 1968; 99: 868
17 Drug Ther Bull 1988; 26: 25
18 J Am Med Ass 1986; 255: 2905
19 Circulation 1977; 56: 385
20 J Cardiov Pharmac 1987; 10: 38

Pharmacokinetic data on corticosteroids

	pKa	logP	Oral abs %	Bio %	Tmax h	Vd l/kg	PrBd %	Met	T½ h	CL ml/min	AU %	Ref
Betamethasone		1.8	good			1.8	64		6-7	180		1
Budesonide		2.3C				4.4	88		2-3	1400		2
Cortisone		2.1							0.5			3
Dexamethasone		1.8	good			1	67-77		2-5	245		4
Fludrocortisone		2.2C	good		1-2		75		0.5			5
Hydrocortisone	5.1	1.6	good		1	0.3-0.5	75-95		1-2	350-400	<1	6
Methylprednisolone	4.6	2.2C				0.7			3	250		7
Prednisolone		1.6	>95	80	1-2	0.4-1.3	65-90		3-4	100-200		8
Triamcinolone		1.2				1.4-2.1			1.4	750-1100		9

Clinical data on corticosteroids

	Dose mg/day	Ther conc mg/l	CSF/Pl	Milk/Pl	T½ RF	T½ HF	Preg Risk Trim	Drug Int	Ref
								As a class:	
Betamethasone	0.5-0.9						S/P	anticoagulants	10
Budesonide	0.4-1.2 inhal								11
Cortisone	25-50					0	S/P	phenytoin	12
Dexamethasone	0.5-9						S/P	phenobarbitone	13
Fludrocortisone	0.1-0.3						S/P	rifampicin	14
Hydrocortisone	10-30					+	S/P	ephedrine	15
Methylprednisolone	4-48						S/P	cardiac glycosides	16
Prednisolone	5-60	0.65		0.13		+	S/P	diuretics	17
Triamcinolone	4-48						S/P	hypoglycaemics	18

References

1 Eur J Clin Pharmac 1983; 25: 643

2 J Chromatogr 1978; 157: 65

3 Med J Aust 1987; 146: 37

4 Eur J Clin Pharmac 1983; 24: 103

5 Analyt Prof Drug Subs 1974; 3: 281

6 Analyt Prof Drug Subs 1983; 12: 277

7 J Pharm Sci 1985; 74: 375

8 Clin Pharmacokinet 1979; 4: 111

9 Clin Pharmac Ther 1986; 39: 313

10 Clin Pharmac Ther 1986; 39: 313

11 Drugs 1984; 28: 485

12 J Org Chem 1986; 51: 4323

13 Br J Clin Pharmac 1981; 12: 434

14 Arzneim Forsch 1971; 21: 1133

15 J Pediat 1984; 105: 799

16 New Engl J Med 1990; 322: 1459

17 Br J Clin Pharmac 1985; 20: 159

18 Eur J Clin Pharmac 1985; 29: 85

Pharmacokinetic data on hormones and their antagonists

	pKa	logP	Oral abs %	Bio %	Tmax h	Vd l/kg	PrBd %	Met	T½ h	CL ml/min	AU %	Ref
Buserelin			nasal	2-3					1-2		67	1
Cyproterone		3.4C	poor		5-10							2
Danazol		4.2C							4-5			3
Dydrogesterone		3.5C			fast							4
Ethinyloestradiol		4.0C	good			2.9	97		13	380		5
Goserelin						0.2	low		4-5	130		6
Hydroxyprogesterone												7
Medroxyprogesterone						0.6	94		36	1260		8
Methyltestosterone		3.9C			1-2				2			9
Mifepristone		4.8C										10
Norethisterone						4	80		10	450		11
Oestradiol		4.0		low	1-3		50	+			<5	12
Progesterone		3.9						+	0.05		low	13
Testosterone		3.3					98	+	0.25		low	14

Clinical data on hormones and their antagonists

	Dose mg/day	Ther conc mg/l	CSF/Pl	Milk/Pl	T½ RF	T½ HF	Preg Risk Trim	Drug Int	Ref
Buserelin	<2 nasal	0.1		low				As a class:	15
Cyproterone	100	0.1-0.15					C/I	alcohol	16
Danazol	200-400						C/I	antihypertensives	17
Dydrogesterone	20-30						C/I	enzyme inducers	18
Ethinyloestradiol							C/I		19
Goserelin	0.1 sc	0.001			+				20
Hydroxyprogesterone	<500/week im						C/I		21
Medroxyprogesterone	2.5-10			0.7			C/I		22
Methyltestosterone	5-80	0.02-0.04					C/I		23
Mifepristone				0.25					24
Norethisterone	5-25						C/I		25
Oestradiol	2						C/I		26
Progesterone	50 im						C/I		27
Testosterone	50 im						C/I		28

References

1 Br Med J 1987; 295: 96
2 Arzneim Forsch 1976; 26: 914
3 J Int Med Res 1977; 5: Suppl 3, 18
4 Martindale 1989; 29th ed, 1397
5 Br J Clin Pharmac 1982; 13: 325
6 Drugs 1991; 41: 254
7 Martindale 1989; 29th ed, 1401
8 Chemotherapia 1986; 5: 159
9 J Pharm Sci 1972; 61: 1746
10 Drugs 1988; 35: 187
11 Br J Clin Pharmac 1978; 24: 448
12 Med Lett 1986; 28: 119
13 Br Med J 1980; 280: 825
14 Br J Derm 1977; 97: 237
15 Lancet 1985; 2: 1236
16 Arzneim Forsch 1973; 23: 1550
17 Scot Med J 1979; 24: 147
18 Lancet 1977; 2: 982
19 Br Med J 1981; 282: 1516
20 Lancet 1983; 2: 415
21 New Eng J Med 1977; 296: 67
22 Contraception 1977; 16: 605
23 J Clin Pharmac 1973; 13: 142
24 Contraception 1987; 36: Suppl, 1
25 Clin Pharmacokinet 1991; 20: 15
26 Lancet 1987; 2: 856
27 Br Med J 1980; 280: 825
28 Drug Ther Bull 1985; 23: 7

Pharmacokinetic data on miscellaneous agents

	pKa	logP	Oral abs %	Bio %	Tmax h	Vd l/kg	PrBd %	Met	T½ h	CL ml/min	AU %	Ref
Amrinone		-0.6C			<3		low		3-12			1
Antipyrine	1.5	0.4				0.5	low		8-12	50		2
Bacitracin			poor						1-2		9-31	3
Bromocriptine	4.9	6.6C	poor		1-2	3	90-96		3	930	<5	4
Carisoprodol		1.7C	fair									5
Cisapride		3.7C										6
Cocaine	8.7	2.3			1-2				<1	2000	10	7
Cyclandelate		4.6C										8
Dantrolen	7.5		poor		4-6				9		low	9
Distigmine			poor									10
Disulfiram		3.9					96		7			11
Dopexamine	*8.6	3.0C			6-9				0.1		low	12
Edrophonium						1.1			1-2	750		13
Enoximone		1.6C		80	0.5-1	0.5	70	+			<5	14
Ethanol		-0.2C	good	16	0.5-1	0.5					<5	15
Flumazenil		1.6C	good			1			<1	700-1200	<0.1	16
Glutethimide	9.2	1.9										17
Levamisole	8.0											18
Lisuride		2.7C		20		19	98		2	750-1500		19
Mefloquin		3.4C	good		2-14				21d	30	5	20
Methocarbamol		-0.1C										21
Misoprostol		2.9C										22
Monosialoganglioside**						0.05-0.09						23
Neostigmine						0.7			1.3	630	67	24
Nizatidine	12.0	-0.6C	>95	95	1-2	1.2	15-30		1.3	840	65	25

Continued on next page

Pharmacokinetic data on miscellaneous agents (Continued)

	pKa	logP	Oral abs %	Bio %	Tmax h	Vd l/kg	PrBd %	Met	T½ h	CL ml/min	AU %	Ref
Ondansetron		3.2C										26
Oxybutynin		3.7C										27
Pamidronate			low						2-3	300	iv 30	28
Papaverine	6.4	3.0C	100	54	1-2		80		1-2		<1	29
Pargyline	6.9	2.0C										30
Pelrinone						16	moderate		1-2		high	31
Pentamidine		2.0C	poor	31	2-3	2.2	low		6.2	8500	<5	32
Pentoxifylline			>90		1-2		90	+	1		<1	33
Pergolide		3.8C			0.5							34
Physostigmine	*1.8	2.2C	sc			1-2	4-18	+	<0.3			35
Pinacidil		1.9C	c100	c95	0.5-1		60-65		4		<10	36
Piracetam		-1.5C										37
Pyridostigmine	7.8	1.2	poor	14		1.1			2-4	640		38
Scopolamine		0.8C										39
Sumatriptan												40
Tacrine		3.3C	poor	<5					2-3	600	<3	41
Tetrahydrocannabinol				10-20	2	10	97	+	>20	760-1190	0	42
Thalidomide		0.3										43
Theobromine	*0.1	-0.8										44
Ticlopidine		4.0C	90		1-2			+			<5	45
Tolrestat			good		2		99.5		10-12		high	46
Tranylcypromine	8.2	1.5	good						2		<2	47
Trazodone			good	81			93		4-7		<1	48
Tubocurarine	*8.0						50		2	160	63	49
Xamoterol		0.5C	9			0.4				140		50
Zimeldine	*3.8	2.7C										51

* = more than one ionizable group ; **GM1 (Svennerholm nomenclature)

Clinical data on miscellaneous agents

	Dose mg/day	Ther conc mg/l	CSF/Pl	Milk/Pl	T½ RF	T½ HF	Preg Risk Trim	Drug Int	Ref
Amrinone									52
Antipyrine	10/kg iv*					+			53
Bacitracin									54
Bromocriptine	10.80	0.001-0.004			0			alcohol	55
Carisoprodol		10-30							56
Cisapride									57
Cocaine									58
Cyclandelate									59
Dantrolen									60
Distigmine	20								61
Disulfiram	100-200	0.4					C/I		62
Dopexamine	0.18/kg inf	100							63
Edrophonium	1 iv	<0.15							64
Enoximone									65
Ethanol		1000		0.8				hypnotics	66
Flumazenil	2 iv	0.05							67
Glutethimide		0.2-0.8							68
Levamisole									69
Lisuride		0.0001							70
Mefloquin	250/w	0.4-1							71
Methocarbamol									72
Misoprostol									73
Monosialoganglioside	100 iv	40							74
Neostigmine					+				75
Nizatidine		0.7			+				76

Continued on next page

Clinical data on miscellaneous agents (Continued)

	Dose mg/day	Ther conc mg/l	CSF/Pl	Milk/Pl	T½ RF	T½ HF	Preg Risk Trim	Drug Int	Ref
Ondansetron									77
Oxybutynin									78
Pamidronate	300-600	2							79
Papaverine		0.6							80
Pargyline									81
Pelrinone	100								82
Pentamidine									83
Pentoxifylline	1200	1		0.9					84
Pergolide	up to 5	1-2							85
Physostigmine									86
Pinacidil									87
Piracetam									88
Pyridostigmine		0.05-0.1			+				89
Scopolamine									90
Sumatriptan			low						91
Tacrine	25-50	0.01							92
Tetrahydrocannabinol	inhal	0.05	low						93
Thalidomide									94
Theobromine									95
Ticlopidine	1000	10-20							96
Tolrestat									97
Tranylcypromine	10-20	0.04						sympathomimetics	98
Trazodone									99
Tubocurarine		0.6-1.2			+				100
Xamoterol									101
Zimeldine									102

References

1 Clin Pharmacokinet 1987; 13: 91
2 Clin Pharmac Ther 1979; 26: 275
3 Ann Int Med 1967; 67: 151
4 Eur J Clin Pharmac 1979; 15: 275
5 Martindale, 29th ed 1990, 1231
6 Drug Dev Res 1986; 8: 225
7 Analyt Prof Drug Subs 1986; 15: 151
8 Arzneim Forsch 1962; 12: 853
9 J Am Med Ass 1975; 231: 862
10 Martindale 29th ed 1990, 1329
11 J Pharm Pharmac 1990; 42: 806
12 Br J Clin Pharmac 1986; 21: 393
13 Clin Pharmac Ther 1976; 19: 813
14 Clin Pharmacokinet 1987; 13: 91
15 Gen Pharmac 1990; 21: 267
16 Br J Clin Pharmac 1986; 22: 421
17 Clin Pharmac Ther 1971; 12: 849
18 Biopharm Drug Disposit 1986; 7: 71
19 Eur J Clin Pharmac 1991; 40: 399
20 Clin Pharmacokinet 1985; 10: 187
21 Martindale 29th ed, 1990, 1235
22 Dig Dis Sci 1985; 30: Suppl 126S
23 Clin Pharmac Ther 1991; 50: 141
24 Anesthesiology 1983; 59: 220
25 Clin Pharmac Ther 1985; 37: 162
26 Eur J Pharmac 1987; 138: 303
27 Therapie 1967; 22: 521
28 Drugs 1991; 41: 289
29 Eur J Clin Pharmac 1984; 27: 127
30 J Pharm Pharmac 1981; 33: 341
31 J Med Chem 1987; 30: 1342
32 J Infect Dis 1985; 152: 750
33 Drugs 1987; 34: 50
34 Clin Neuropharmac 1985; 8: 131
35 J Pharm Pharmac 1990; 42: 804
36 Clin Pharmac Ther 1986; 40: 650
37 J Pharm Belg 1972; 27: 281
38 Eur J Clin Pharmac 1980; 18: 423

39 J Pharm Sci 1984; 73: 561
40 Br J Pharmac 1988; 94: 1123
41 Clin Pharmac Ther 1989; 43: 634
42 Med Res Rev 1983; 3: 119
43 Proc Nat Acad Sci 1981; 78: 2545
44 Clin Pharmac Ther 1983; 34: 546
45 Drugs 1987; 34: 222
46 Clin Pharmac Ther 1984; 36: 493
47 Clin Pharmac Ther 1986; 40: 444
48 Br J Clin Pharmac 1983; 16: 371
49 Clin Pharmacokinet 1977; 2: 230
50 Drug Met Dispos 1984; 12: 652
51 Arzneim Forsch 1981; 31: 486
52 New Engl J Med 1986; 314: 349
53 Br J Clin Pharmac 1984; 18: 559
54 Antimicrob Ag Chemother 1984; 25: 502
55 Ann Intern Med 1984; 100: 78
56 Martindale, 29th ed, 1231
57 Drug Dev Res 1986; 8: 251
58 Science 1978; 200: 211
59 Arzneim Forsch 1957; 7: 15
60 Drugs 1986; 32: 130
61 Arzneim Forsch 1968; 18: 479
62 Clin Pharmac Ther 1984; 36: 520
63 Eur J Clin Pharmac 1987; 32: 1
64 Br J Anaesthes 1986; 58: 825
65 Drugs of Today 1990; 26: 373
66 Clin Pharmacokinet 1980; 5: 1
67 J Clin Pharmac 1985; 25: 400
68 New Engl J Med 1975; 292: 250
69 Eur J Drug Met Pharmacokinet 1982; 7: 247
70 Eur Neurol 1983; 22: 240
71 Eur J Clin Pharmac 1987; 32: 173
72 Clin Med 1966; 73: 41
73 Drugs 1987; 33: 1
74 Stroke 1989; 20: 1143
75 Anesthesiology 1979; 51: 222
76 Am J Gastroent 1986; 81: 1167
77 Cancer Treat Rev 1987; 14: 333
78 New Engl J Med 1985; 313: 800
79 J Nucl Med 1985; 26: 1135

References

1 Eur J Clin Pharmac 1989; 37: 525
2 Clin Pharmac Ther 1978; 23: 585
3 Drug Met Rev 1975; 4: 267
4 Drugs 1975; 10: 241
5 Eur J Clin Pharmac 1980; 18: 355
6 J Am Pharm Ass Sci Ed 1953; 42: 457
7 Analyt Prof Drug Subs 1973; 2: 295
8 J Clin Pharmac 1972; 12: 453
9 Eur J Clin Pharmac 1985; 28: 89
10 Br J Clin Pharmac 1979; 8: 459
11 Drugs 1985; 29: 342
12 J Pharmacokinet Biopharm 1973; 1: 319
13 Clin Pharmac Ther 1986; 40: 444
14 Clin Pharmac Ther 1983; 33: 355
15 Eur J Clin Pharmac 1984; 27: 123
16 Curr Med Res Opin 1979; 6: Suppl 1, 107
17 Curr Med Res opin 1979; 6: Suppl 1, 15
18 Br J Clin Pharmac 1977; 4: 648P
19 Therapie 1984; 39: 509
20 Med Lett 1986; 28: 51
21 Acta Neurol Scand 1979; 60: 250
22 Int Clin Psychopharmac 1987; 2: 165
23 Curr Ther Res 1980; 27: 429
24 Med J Aust 1987; 146: 634
25 Pharmacotherapeutica 1983; 3: 300
26 Arch Gen Psychiat 1985; 42: 962

Pharmacokinetic data on monoamine-oxidase inhibitors and appetite suppressants

	pKa	logP	Oral abs %	Bio %	Tmax h	Vd l/kg	PrBd %	Met	T½ h	CL ml/min	AU %	Ref
Caffeine	* 0.6	-0.1	good						3-5			1
Dexamphetamine	9.9	1.8	good			3-4	15-40	+	4-12		1-75	2
Diethylpropion		2.5C	good					+	1.5-3		<1	3
Fenfluramine	9.1	3.4	good		2-4		30-35	+	11-30		2-23	4
Flupenthixol	7.8	4.5	good	55	3-6	12-17			14-36	500		5
Iproniazid	10.4	0.2C	good						10		15	6
Isocarboxazid		1.5	good					+	36		2	7
Mazindol	8.6								36		12-24	8
Moclobemide	10.5	2.1C		60					1-2			9
Pemoline			good		2-3		30-50		10-18		50	10
Phenelzine		0.9C	good						7		<5	11
Phentermine	10.1	1.9	good		4	3-4			19-24		70-80	12
Tranylcypromine	8.2	1.5	good						2		<2	13

* = more than one ionizable group

Clinical data on monoamine-oxidase inhibitors and appetite suppressants

	Dose mg/day	Ther conc mg/l	CSF/Pl	Milk/Pl	T½ RF	T½ HF	Preg Risk Trim	Drug Int	Ref
Caffeine				c2,avoid					14
Dexamphetamine	10-60	<0.1		avoid				other MAOIs	15
Diethylpropion	75	0.007						sympathomimetics	16
Fenfluramine	60-120	0.05-0.15	+					alcohol	17
Flupenthixol	0.5-3						S/P	anticonvulsants	18
Iproniazid	25-150								19
Isocarboxazid	10-30							narcotic analgesics	20
Mazindol	2							antidepressants	21
Moclobemide	200	1							22
Pemoline	40-120	0.8-1.2						other MAOIs	23
Phenelzine	45-60	0.002-0.05						antidepressants	24
Phentermine	15-30	0.1						alcohol	25
Tranylcypromine	10-20	0.04						sympathomimetics	26

References *(continued)*

80 Br Med J 1987; 295: 595
81 J Am Med Ass 1967; 201: 57
82 J Med Chem 1988; 31: 814
83 Rev Infect Dis 1985; 7: 625
84 Angiology 1986; 37: 555
85 Neurology 1985; 35: 296
86 New Engl J Med 1983; 308: 721
87 Clin Pharmac Ther 1987; 42: 50
88 J Clin Psychopharmac 1985; 5: 272
89 Clin Pharmac Ther 1980; 28: 78
90 Br J Clin Pharmac 1983; 16: 623
91 Lancet 1988; 1: 1309
92 Age Ageing 1989; 18: 223
93 Br Med J 1987; 294: 141
94 Br J Dermatol 1985; 112: 475
95 Clin Pharmac Ther 1977; 21: 115
96 Drugs 1986; 31: 517
97 Clin Pharmac Ther 1985; 38: 625
98 Arch Dis Psychiat 1985; 42: 962
99 Drugs 1981; 21: 401
100 Br J Anaesthes 1980; 52: 893
101 Br J Clin Pharmac 1986; 22: 595
102 Drugs 1982; 24: 169

Pharmacokinetic data on penicillins

	pKa	logP	Oral abs %	Bio %	Tmax h	Vd l/kg	PrBd %	Met	T½ h	CL ml/min	AU %	Ref
Amoxycillin	*2.4	0.3C	good		1-2	0.2-0.4	20		1	200-400	50-70	1
Ampicillin	*2.5	0.6	fair		2	0.2-0.5	20		1-2	200-280	30-90	2
Azlocillin	*2.8		poor			0.2	30		1	150	50-60	3
Bacampicillin	*6.8	2.0C	65		0.5-1			+a			low	4
Bacmecillinam					1				1		41b	5
Benzylpenicillin	*2.8	1.8	30		1	0.4	45-65		0.5-1	500	20-85	6
Carbenicillin	*2.6	1.1	poor			0.2	50		1.2	130	80-85	7
Ciclacillin			good		0.5-1		20-25		0.5		60-70	8
Cloxacillin	*2.8	2.4	var			0.1	94		0.3-2	200	35-65	9
Dicloxacillin	*2.7	2.9	good			0.2	98		0.8	130	35-70	10
Flucloxacillin	*2.7		good		1	0.15	93	+	1.5	83		11
Mecillinam	*3.4		poor			0.4	5-15		1		50-70	12
Methicillin	*2.8	1.2	poor			0.4	40		0.6	500	25-80	13
Mezlocillin			poor			0.25	35		1	200	60-70	14
Phenethicillin	*2.7	2.2	var	86	2	0.3	75		1	295	50	15
PhenoxyMepenicillin	*2.7		good	50	2	0.5	80		0.5	480	20-35	16
Piperacillin			poor			0.2	22		1	166	75-90	17
Pivampicillin	*7.0	2.4C	good		1			+a			low	18
Pivmecillinam	*8.9		good		1-2			+b	0.7		30b	19
Sultamicillin		1.7C	good					+a				20
Talampicillin		1.2C	good		0.5-1			+a				21
Ticarcillin	*2.5	1.2C	poor			0.2	60		1.2	140	80-90	22

* = more than one ionizable group ; a = ampicillin ; b = mecillinam

Clinical data on penicillins

	Dose mg/day	Ther conc mg/l	CSF/Pl	Milk/Pl	T½ RF	T½ HF	Preg Risk Trim	Drug Int	Ref
Amoxycillin	750-1500	6-15	+		+				23
Ampicillin	1000-8000	7-14		low	+				24
Azlocillin	2000-6000iv			low					25
Bacampicillin	800-2400								26
Bacmecillinam	1200-1600	2-4							27
Benzylpenicillin	600-2400	12		0.4	+				28
Carbenicillin	1000-2000im	50		<0.001	+	+			29
Ciclacillin	1000-2000				+				30
Cloxacillin	2000	7-14		+	0				31
Dicloxacillin	500	10-18			0				32
Flucloxacillin	1000-2000	5-15			+				33
Mecillinam	400 im	6-12	low	low	+				34
Methicillin	<12000 iv	10	low	low	+				35
Mezlocillin	6000-8000iv	45	low	low	+	+			36
Phenethicillin	1000-2000								37
PhenoxyMepenicillin	500-3000	3-6							38
Piperacillin	<20000 iv	30-40			+				39
Pivampicillin	1000-2000								40
Pivmecillinam	1200-1600	5							41
Sultamicillin	250								42
Talampicillin	750-1500								43
Ticarcillin	<20000 iv	20-30			+				44

References

1 Drugs 1979; 18: 169
2 Clin Pharmacokinet 1976; 1: 297
3 J Antimicrob Chemother 1983;
11: B101
4 J Antimicrob Chemother 1981; 8:
Suppl C41
5 Eur J Clin Pharmac 1982; 23: 249
6 Clin Pharmacokinet 1976; 1: 297
7 Antimicrob Ag Chemother 1980;
17: 608
8 Antimicrob Ag Chemother 1981;
19: 1086
9 J Paedriatr 1984; 105: 829
10 Antimicrob Ag Chemother 1976;
10: 441
11 Eur J Clin Pharmac 1985; 27:
713
12 Antimicrob Ag Chemother 1983;
23: 827
13 Rev Infect Dis 1985; 7: 287
14 J Antimicrob Chemother 1983;
11: Suppl C 1
15 Br J Clin Pharmac 1985; 19: 657
16 Br J Clin Pharmac 1985; 19: 657
17 Drugs 1984; 28: 375
18 J Antimicrob Chemother 1975; 1:
39
19 Eur J Clin Pharmac 1982; 23:
249
20 J Antimicrob Chemother 1982;
10: 49
21 Drugs of Today 1979; 15: 349
22 J Int Med Res 1977; 5: 308
23 Drugs 1981; 22: 337
24 Clin Pharmac Ther 1983; 34: 792
25 Ann Intern Med 1982; 97: 755
26 Pharmacotherapy 1982; 2: 313
27 Lymphology 1979; 12: 85
28 Drugs 1986; 31: 266
29 Eur J Resp Dis 1986; 69: 160
30 Am J Kid Dis 1983; 3: 155
31 Br Med J 1987; 294: 42
32 Drug Intell Clin Pharm 1984; 18:
530
33 Eur J Clin Pharmac 1987; 32:
403
34 Pharmacotherapy 1985; 5: 1
35 Antimicrob Ag Chemother 1978;
14: 723
36 Antimicrob Ag Chemother 1984;
25: 556
37 Br J Clin Pharmac 1985; 19: 657
38 Lancet 1982; 2: 140
39 J Antimicrob Chemother 1982; 9:
489
40 Drug Ther Bull 1981; 19: 78
41 Antimicrob Ag Chemother 1978;
13: 90
42 J Antimicrob Chemother 1982;
10: 49
43 Br J Vener Dis 1982; 58: 180
44 J Antimicrob Chemother 1987;
19: 363

Pharmacokinetic data on quinolone antibiotics

	pKa	logP	Oral abs %	Bio %	Tmax h	Vd l/kg	PrBd %	Met	T½ h	CL ml/min	AU %	Ref
Acrosoxacin	*8.1	0.7			3-4		70		3-11		<5	1
Amifloxacin					1				4		54	2
Cinoxacin	*4.7	-2.0	c100		6	0.25	16-60		2-4	210	50-60	3
Ciprofloxacin	*6.0	-1.6	c100	70	1	3	20-40	+	3-6	500	30-50	4
Enoxacin	*6.0	-2.0	good	80	1-3	2.3	20-60		3-6	350	30-50	5
Lomefloxacin			c100	c100	1				7-8	200-300	10-20	6
Nalidixic acid	*6.7	-2.0	c100		1-2	1	93-95	+	2-9	160	<20	7
Norfloxacin	*6.3	-1.4		40	1-2	2	15		3-4		30	8
Ofloxacin		-2.0	c100	90	1-2	1.2	20-30	+	4-7	560	85-95	9
Pefloxacin		-1.5	c100	95	1-3	1.8	20-30	+	8-15	150	<10	10

* = more than one ionizable group

Clinical data on quinolone antibiotics

	Dose mg/day	Ther conc mg/l	CSF/Pl	Milk/Pl	T½ RF	T½ HF	Preg Risk Trim	Drug Int	Ref
Acrosoxacin	300						S/P		11
Amifloxacin	2400	8			+				12
Cinoxacin	1000	15			0		C/I		13
Ciprofloxacin	500-1500	2-3	low		0	+	C/I	theophylline	14
Enoxacin	200-600	1-4			+		C/I		15
Lomefloxacin	200-800	1-2			+				16
Nalidixic acid	2000-4000	20-50			avoid		C/I	anticoagulants	17
Norfloxacin	400	1-2			+		C/I		18
Ofloxacin	200-400	2-6			+		C/I	theophylline	19
Pefloxacin	400-1200	1-10	<1		0	+	C/I	theophylline	20

References

1 Invest Urol 1979; 17: 149
2 Antimicrob Ag Chemother 1985; 27: 774
3 Antimicrob Ag Chemother 1979; 15: 165
4 Antimicrob Ag Chemother 1987; 31: 956
5 J Antimicrob Chemother 1986; 18: Suppl D, 7
6 Biopharm Drug Disposit 1990; 11: 543
7 J Clin Pharmac 1982; 22: 490
8 J Antimicrob Chemother 1984; 13: Suppl B, 59
9 Drugs 1987; 34: Suppl 1, 21
10 Drugs 1989; 37: 628
11 Antimicrob Ag Chemother 1980; 18: 738
12 Drugs of the Future 1990; 15: 282
13 Clin Pharmac Ther 1976; 19: 119
14 Chemotherapy 1990; 36: 385
15 J Antimicrob Chemother 1984; 14: Suppl C, 1
16 Antimicrob Ag Chemother 1988; 32: 617
17 New Engl J Med 1991; 324: 384
18 Drugs 1985; 30: 482
19 Am J Med 1989; 87: Suppl 5A, 24
20 Eur J Clin Microb 1987; 6: 521

Pharmacokinetic data on respiratory agents

	pKa	logP	Oral abs %	Bio %	Tmax h	Vd l/kg	PrBd %	Met	T½ h	CL ml/min	AU %	Ref
Acetylcysteine	9.5	-0.6C	good		1-3	0.4	64-78		6	slow		1
Adrenaline	*8.7	-1.4	poor	0			50				<1	2
Astemazole		4.1	good			250	>95		20			3
Beclomethasone		4.2C	good						15			4
Betamethasone		1.8	good			1.8	64		6-7	180		5
Bromhexine	8.5	4.9C	good		0.5-3				6		<1	6
Brompheniramine	*9.2	0.2			3			+	15		10	7
Budesonide		2.3C				4.4	88		2-3	1400		8
Carbocisteine		-2.6C			2-4				1	530		9
Chlorpheniramine	*9.1	3.4	c100	35	2-3	3	70		18-40	100	3-10	10
Clemastine		5.1C			3-5							11
Codeine	8.2	1.1	good	50	0.5-2	3.5-5	7-25	+	2-4	700-1600	6-16	12
Cyproheptadine	8.9	4.7			6-9						5	13
Dextromethorphan	8.3	4.0C	good			2					<10	14
Diamorphine	7.6	1.0	good			3-5	20-35	+	0.05	1000-1400	<1	15
Diphenhydramine	9.0	3.3	good	50	2-4	4-8	80-98		5-9	700	<5	16
Diphenylpyraline	9.1	3.4C	good						20-40		<10	17
Doxapram		3.1C	good	60		3			7	350		18
Ephedrine	9.6	1.0	good					+	3-11		50-75	19
Fenoterol	*8.5	0.8C	60	low	2				6-7		<2	20

Continued on next page

Pharmacokinetic data on respiratory agents (Continued)

	pKa	logP	Oral abs %	Bio %	Tmax h	Vd l/kg	PrBd %	Met	T½ h	CL ml/min	AU %	Ref
Hydroxyzine	*7.1	4.2C			2-4				3			21
Ipratropium			inhal	<1					3-4		low	22
Isoprenaline	*8.6	0.1C	irreg		1-2	0.5	68		0.05		<5	23
Mepyramine	*8.9	0.5						+				24
Methadone	8.3	2.1	good	30	4	5	80-90		10-25	140	33	25
Noscapine	6.2	2.5C	good	40	0.5-2	3-7			1.5-3	1400	<1	26
Orciprenaline	*10.0	0.7	good		1-3				2			27
Phenindamine	8.3	2.0C										28
Pheniramine	*9.3	0.8C			1-3				8-17			29
Pholcodine	*8.0	-0.5C			5				37			30
Pirbuterol	*7.0	2.9			2				2-3		10	31
Promethazine	9.1	-0.9C	>80	25	2	13	75-93		10-15	1120	2	32
Reproterol												33
Rimiterol	*8.7	0.2C	good	low	1-3				<0.1		10	34
Salbutamol	*9.3	0.1C	90		0.25		low		2-7		50	35
Sodium cromoglycate	*2.5	1.9	poor		2-4		60-70		1-2	560	<5	36
Terbutaline	*8.7	0.5C		c15	0.5-2	1	15-25		3-15	200-300	10	37
Theophylline	*8.6	-0.0			4-7	0.5	40-50	+	3-13	35-140	7-13	38
Trimeprazine	*9.0	4.6C	good		2							39
Tripolidine	*6.9	3.9							1.5-2			40

* = more than one ionizable group

Clinical data on respiratory agents

	Dose mg/day	Ther conc mg/l	CSF/Pl	Milk/Pl	T½ RF	T½ HF	Preg Risk Trim	Drug Int	Ref
Acetylcysteine	600	0.4-4							41
Adrenaline	0.2-0.5sc							maois	42
Astemazole	10-30		low						43
Beclomethasone	0.3-0.4 inhal						C/I		44
Betamethasone	0.6-0.8 inhal						S/P		45
Bromhexine	24-64	0.01-0.14							46
Brompheniramine	12-32	0.012-0.017							47
Budesonide	0.4-1.2 inhal								48
Carbocisteine	1500	8							49
Chlorpheniramine	12-16	0.01-0.04			0			alcohol	50
Clemastine	2	0.002		avoid					51
Codeine	45-120	0.11-0.23		2.2	0			maois	52
Cyproheptadine	32							alcohol	53
Dextromethorphan	40-50	0.001-0.008							54
Diamorphine	9-36	*							55
Diphenhydramine	75	0.1-1			+			cns depressants	56
Diphenylpyraline	10-20								57
Doxapram									58
Ephedrine	45-180	0.04-0.14						tricyclics	59
Fenoterol	0.2-0.4 inhal						3	sympathomimetics	60

Continued on next page

* = metabolised to morphine

Clinical data on respiratory agents (Continued)

	Dose mg/day	Ther conc mg/l	CSF/Pl	Milk/Pl	T½ RF	T½ HF	Preg Risk Trim	Drug Int	Ref
Hydroxyzine	200-400	0.07-0.09					C/I		61
Ipratropium	0.04 inhal								62
Isoprenaline	30-60 sl							anaesthetics	63
Mepyramine	300								64
Methadone	6-12	0.05-1		0.5	+			cns depressants	65
Noscapine									66
Orciprenaline	80	0.002-0.01						tricyclics	67
Phenindamine	100-200								68
Pheniramine	150	0.01-0.19							69
Pholcodine	60	0.02							70
Pirbuterol	30-60								71
Promethazine	20-75	0.01					S/P		72
Reproterol	30-60								73
Rimiterol	0.2-0.5 inhal	0.001							74
Salbutamol	6-32	0.1					3	sympathomimetics	75
Sodium cromoglycate	8-16 inhal	0.006-0.012						maois	76
Terbutaline	1-15	0.002-0.005		1			3	sympathomimetics	77
Theophylline	180-1000	10-15		c1,avoid	0		3	cimetidine	78
Trimeprazine	30-40	0.0008-0.002							79
Tripolidine	7.5-15	0.004-0.017		0.53					80

References

1 Clin Pharmacokinet 1991; 20: 123
2 J Pharm Sci 1977; 66: 447
3 Drugs 1984; 28: 38
4 Med J Aust 1987; 146: 37
5 Eur J Clin Pharmac 1983; 25: 643
6 Biopharm Drug Disposit 1982; 3: 337
7 Br J Clin Pharmac 1982; 14: 49
8 Arzneim Forsch 1979; 29: 1687
9 Eur J Clin Pharmac 1991; 40: 387
10 Analyt Prof Drug Subs 1973; 7: 43
11 Arzneim Forsch 1978; 28: 1017
12 Clin Pharmac Ther 1978; 24: 60
13 Analyt Prof Drug Subs 1980; 9: 155
14 J Pharm Sci 1977; 66: 1047
15 Drug Met Rev 1975; 4: 39
16 Clin Pharmac Ther 1974; 16: 1066
17 J Pharmacokinet Biopharm 1974; 2: 191
18 Br J Clin Pharmac 1979; 7: 81
19 Br J Clin Pharmac 1976; 3: 123
20 Drugs 1978; 15: 3
21 J Pharm Sci 1979; 68: 1456
22 Postgrad Med J 1975; 51: Suppl 7, 76
23 Br J Pharmac 1972; 46: 958
24 J Pharm Sci 1976; 65: 612
25 Clin Pharmacokinet 1986; 11: 87
26 Analyt Prof Drug Subs 1982; 11: 407
27 Arzneim Forsch 1979; 29: 967
28 Int J Clin Pharmac Ther Tox 1985; 23: 59
29 J Analyt Toxicol 1979; 3: 253
30 Br J Clin Pharmac 1986; 22: 61
31 Drugs 1985; 30: 6
32 Br J Clin Pharmac 1983; 15: 287
33 Arzneim Forsch 1978; 28: 765
34 Br J Clin Pharmac 1976; 3: 583
35 Br J Clin Pharmac 1986; 22: 587
36 J Pharm Pharmac 1978; 30: 386
37 Br J Clin Pharmac 1974; 1: 129
38 Drug Met Rev 1983; 14: 295
39 J Chromatogr 1982; 233: 417
40 J Pharm Sci 1977; 66: 841
41 Drugs 1983; 25: 290
42 Drugs 1985; 30: 552
43 Arzneim Forsch 1983; 33: 381
44 Drug Ther Bull 1986; 24: 1
45 Clin Pharmac Ther 1986; 39: 313
46 Clin Tr J 1983; 20: 115
47 New Engl J Med 1975; 293: 486
48 Drugs 1984; 28: 485
49 Lancet 1990; 335: 1107
50 New Engl J Med 1983; 308: 1275
51 Lancet 1982; 1: 914
52 J Int Med Res 1983; 11: 92
53 Drug Met Disposit 1975; 3: 1
54 Lancet 1984; 2: 517
55 Lancet 1984; 1: 1449
56 Clin Pharmac Ther 1974; 16: 1066
57 J Forens Sci 1974; 19: 193
58 Br J Clin Pharmac 1981; 11: 305
59 Br J Clin Pharmac 1975; 2: 180P
60 Clin Pharm 1985; 4: 393
61 Analyt Prof Drug Subs 1978; 7: 319
62 New Engl J Med 1988; 319: 486
63 J Am Med Ass 1986; 255: 2905
64 Clin Toxicol 1981; 18: 907
65 New Engl J Med 1987; 317: 447
66 Eur J Clin Pharmac 1982; 22: 535
67 Ann Intern Med 1980; 93: 428
68 J Forens Sci 1974; 19: 193
69 Int J Clin Pharmac Ther Tox 1985; 23: 59
70 J Clin Pharm Ther 1988; 13: 5
71 Drug Ther Bull 1984; 22: 70
72 Br Med J 1985; 290: 1173
73 Clin Ter (Rome) 1981; 98: 481
74 Clin Tr J 1973; 10: 13
75 Br Med J 1984; 288: 1595
76 Lancet 1986; 1: 242
77 Arzneim Forsch 1982; 32: 159

References *(continued)*

78 Prescribers J 1986; 26: 26

79 Br J Clin Pharmac 1983; 15:
   604P

80 Curr Ther Res 1980; 28: 650

Pharmacokinetic data on sulphonamides and other antibacterials

	pKa	logP	Oral abs %	Bio %	Tmax h	Vd l/kg	PrBd %	Met	T½ h	CL ml/min	AU %	Ref
Chloramphenicol	* 5.5	1.1	good		1-2	0.5-1	40-60		2-5	200-300	5-10	1
Clindamycin	7.7	2.2	90		1	0.8	93		3	200	5-15	2
Colistin			poor		2-3				2-5		80	3
Erythromycin	8.9	2.5	var		2	0.7	70-80		1-3	400-500	5-15	4
Fusidic acid	5.4	5.6C			2-3	0.5	95	+	5-6		<10	5
Lincomycin	7.5	0.6	20-35		2-4	0.8	72		5		10-15	6
Nitrofurantoin	7.2						40		1	680		7
Polymyxin B	8.9		0		2				6		60	8
Roxithromycin					1		86-91		13	23	<5	9
Spectinomycin	* 8.7	-2.5C			1	0.2	low		2	100	35-90	10
Sulfametopyrazine			good				60-80		c50		<20	11
Sulfaurea			good						2-3			12
Sulphadiazine	* 6.5	-0.1	good		4	0.3	20-50		6-17**	25	<50	13
Sulphadimidine	7.4	2.0	good		3-4	0.2-0.6	60-90		1-11**	30	<15	14
Sulphaguanidine	* 2.8	-1.2	var				<10					15
Sulphamethoxazole	5.6	0.9	good		2-4	0.2	60-70		9-12	15-25	60-80	16
Thiamphenicol		-0.3							2			17
Trimethoprim	7.2	0.9	c100		1-4	1.4	40-70		8-17	75-150	40-70	18
Vancomycin			poor			0.4-1	10-55		4-10	75	90-100	19

* = more than one ionizable group   ** = genetic polymorphism

Clinical data on sulphonamides and other antibacterials

	Dose mg/day	Ther conc mg/l	CSF/Pl	Milk/Pl	T½ RF	T½ HF	Preg Risk Trim	Drug Int	Ref
Chloramphenicol	2000	10-20	+	cl,avoid	0	+	3	anticoagulants	20
Clindamycin	600-1200	0.5		0.3	+	+		neuromusc blockers	21
Colistin	6 mega-units	1-5	0	+	+				22
Erythromycin	1000-4000	2-6	0	0.4	+			theophylline	23
Fusidic acid	1500	30		+	0		C/I		24
Lincomycin	1500-2000	1-3		+	+			neuromusc blockers	25
Nitrofurantoin	300			0.1					26
Polymyxin B	180000 units		0				C/I	nephrotoxins	27
Roxithromycin	300	9							28
Spectinomycin	2000 im	100							29
Sulfametopyrazine	2000 weekly				0		3		30
Sulfaurea	3000		+				3	hypoglycaemics	31
Sulphadiazine	6000-9000	19-40					3		32
Sulphadimidine	2000-4000	50-100			+		3,C/I	frusimide	33
Sulphaguanidine	9000-12000	15-40					3		34
Sulphamethoxazole	2000-3000	28-45			+		C/I	folate inhibitors	35
Thiamphenicol									36
Trimethoprim	400	3-10			+		1,C/I		37
Vancomycin	500-2000iv	10-40			+	+			38

References

1 Clin Pharmacokinet 1984; 9: 222
2 J Clin Pharmac 1972; 12: 74
3 Medicamenta 1973; 61: 177
4 J Clin Pharmac 1982; 22: 321
5 J Antimicrob Chemother 1987; 20: 467
6 Clin Pharmac Ther 1971; 12: 793
7 Clin Pharmac Ther 1981; 29: 808
8 J Antimicrob Chemother 1986; 17: 333
9 Antimicrob Ag Chemother 1987; 31: 1051
10 Drugs 1972; 3: 314
11 J Antimicrob Chemother 1980; 6: 647
12 Martindale 1989; 29th edn, 310
13 Clin Pharmacokinet 1980; 5: 274
14 Clin Pharmacokinet 1980; 5: 274
15 Martindale 1989; 29th edn, 305
16 Clin Pharmacokinet 1978; 3: 319
17 Antimicrob Ag Chemother 1976; 9: 557
18 J Int Med Res 1983; 11: 137
19 Clin Pharmacokinet 1983; 2: 417
20 Antimicrob Ag Chemother 1979; 15: 651
21 Antimicrob Ag Chemother 1975; 7: 153
22 Drug Intell Clin Pharm 1970; 4: 332
23 J Antimicrob Chemother 1986; 18: 293
24 Br Med J 1977; 2: 36
25 Am J Kid Dis 1983; 3: 155
26 Develop Pharmac Ther 1990; 14: 148
27 Antimicrob Ag Chemother 1977; 12: 655
28 J Antimicrob Chemother 1987; 20: Suppl B, 157
29 Br Med J 1984; 289: 1032
30 Eur J Clin Pharmac 1984; 27: 345
31 Martindale 1989; 29th edn, 310
32 Circulation 1984; 70: 1118A
33 Lancet 1972; 2: 210
34 Martindale 1989; 29th edn, 305
35 Clin Pharmacokinet 1980; 5: 405
36 Eur J Obs Gyn Rep Biol 1977; 7: 383
37 Drugs 1982; 23: 405
38 Br Med J 1982; 284: 1508

Pharmacokinetic data on tetracyclines, aminoglycosides and related agents

	pKa	logP	Oral abs %	Bio %	Tmax h	Vd l/kg	PrBd %	Met	T½ h	CL ml/min	AU %	Ref
Chlortetracycline	* 3.3	-0.9	good			1.2	47-55		6		15	1
Clomocycline		-1.9C			2-3				6		30	2
Demeclocycline	* 3.3	-0.6	good			1.8	40-90		10-15			3
Doxycycline	* 3.5	-0.2	>95		2	0.7	82-90		16-22	28	30-40	4
Lymecycline												5
Minocycline	* 2.8	-1.4C				1.5	70		15	120	<10	6
Oxytetracycline	* 3.3	-1.4C			2-3	1.5	20-35		9		70	7
Tetracycline	* 3.3	-2.6C				1.3-2	25-65		6-9	150-250	20-50	8
Amikacin			poor			0.2	<10		2-3	75	>90	9
Fosfomycin									3	63		10
Gentamicin	8.2		poor			0.2	<30		2-4	75	80-98	11
Kanamycin	7.2		poor			0.3	<5		2-4	100	50-95	12
Neomycin			<5						2-3			13
Netilmicin						0.25	<25		3	67	90-95	14
Tobramycin	* 6.7		poor			0.3	<10		2-3	60-100	90-98	15

* = more than one ionizable group

Clinical data on tetracyclines, aminoglycosides and related agents

	Dose mg/day	Ther conc mg/l	CSF/Pl	Milk/Pl	T½ RF	T½ HF	Preg Risk Trim	Drug Int	Ref
Chlortetracycline	1000-2000						C/I	As a class:	16
Clomocycline	510-1360	1-2					C/I	antacids	17
Demeclocycline	600	2-3					C/I	oral contraceptives	18
Doxycycline	50-100	1.5-3			0		C/I		19
Lymecycline	300	1.4	+				C/I		20
Minocycline	100-200	1-4			0		C/I		21
Oxytetracycline	1000-2000	1.2-3.4			+		C/I		22
Tertacycline	1000-2000	1-5	low	0.6	+		C/I		23
Amikacin	1000 im	15-25		0	+		2,3	As a class:	24
Fosfomycin	2500	40							25
Gentamicin	140-350 im	4-10	low		+		2,3	frusemide	26
Kanamycin	1000 im	20-25	low	low	+		2,3	anaesthetics	27
Neomycin	6000	4-10					2,3	ethacrynic acid	28
Netilmicin	280-420 im	4			+		C/I		29
Tobramycin	210-350 im	4-10	low	+	+		C/I		30

References

1 Drug Intell Clin Pharm 1970; 4: 332
2 Br J Clin Pract 1968; 22: 37
3 New Engl J Med 1985; 312: 1121
4 Ther Drug Monit 1982; 4: 115
5 Br J Clin Pharmac 1984; 18: 529
6 Clin Pharmac Ther 1978; 24: 233
7 J Antimicrob Chemother 1977; 3: 247
8 Drugs 1976; 11: 45
9 Can J Hosp Pharm 1977; 30: 146
10 Antimicrob Ag Chemother 1984; 25: 458
11 Clin Pharmac Ther 1983; 34: 644
12 Clin Pharmacokinet 1979; 4: 170
13 Clin Pharmacokinet 1979; 4: 170
14 Clin Pharmac Ther 1983; 34: 644
15 Eur J Clin Pharmac 1983; 24: 643
16 Acta Odontol Scand 1985; 43: 47
17 Br J Derm 1976; 95: 317
18 J Am Med Ass 1980; 243: 2513
19 Br J Clin Pharmac 1983; 16: 245
20 J Antimicrob Chemother 1978; 4: 187
21 Clin Pharmac Ther 1973; 14: 852
22 Can Med Ass J 1968; 99: 849
23 Mayo Clin Proc 1987; 62: 906
24 Ann Intern Med 1981; 95: 328
25 Br J Clin Pharmac 1984; 17: 477
26 Clin Pharmacokinet 1979; 4: 170
27 Antimicrob Ag Chemother 1981; 20: 515
28 Ann Intern Med 1983; 98: 171
29 J Antimicrob Chemother 1987; 31: 605
30 Drug Ther Bull 1982; 20: 11

Pharmacokinetic data on thyroid and antithyroid agents

	pKa	logP	Oral abs %	Bio %	Tmax h	Vd l/kg	PrBd %	Met	T½ h	CL ml/min	AU %	Ref
Carbimazole				low	1-3		low	+				1
Liothyronine	8.5	3.0C	c100			0.5	99		2d	17		2
Methimazole		0.1C	c100			0.5	low		3-5	170	7-12	3
Propylthiouracil	8.3		c100		1	0.4	80		1-2	120-280	<20	4
Thyroxine	* 2.2		var			0.2	99.9	+	6-7d	2		5

* = more than one ionizable group

Clinical data on thyroid and antithyroid agents

	Dose mg/day	Ther conc mg/l	CSF/Pl	Milk/Pl	T½ RF	T½ HF	Preg Risk Trim	Drug Int	Ref
Carbimazole	30-60	0.5-3.4		avoid					6
Liothyronine	0.1	0.001-0.002						anticoagulants	7
Methimazole					+				8
Propylthiouracil	200-600	1.6-7.5		0.2	+				9
Thyroxine	0.05-0.3	0.05-0.12						phenytoin	10

Index

Two numbers generally appear after each drug, the first referring to the pharmacokinetic and the second the clinical data. In a few cases compounds which are used in several different therapeutic categories are listed in more than one location to permit moɪ rapid comparison with related drugs.